Happy Life at a
Healthy Weight

Happy Life at a Healthy Weight

Creating a Shame Free, Healthy Relationship with Food and Life

Kay Loughrey RDN, MPH

Published by Authentic Wellness Publishing Company, LLC

ISBN (paperback): 979-8-9910260-0-0
ISBN (ebook): 979-8-9910260-1-7

Book design and production by www.AuthorSuccess.com
Cover art by www.istockphoto.com

Please note:
The information and recommendations in this book are offered for educational purposes only and are not intended to provide medical advice, nutrition counseling/medical nutrition therapy, or psychotherapy. Please see your health provider, registered dietitian-nutritionist, or a mental health professional if you have diet-related medical conditions or mental health conditions such as depression, anxiety, or an eating disorder.

I dedicate this book to my late husband, Jacob.
This book is a testament to your unwavering
faith in my dreams and the love we shared.

Contents

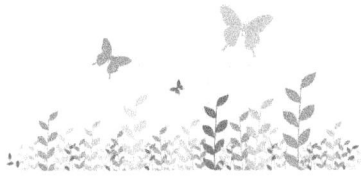

Introduction

JULIE CALLED ME ONE DAY because she was frustrated with dieting and her weight. She said, "I was 140 pounds when I started dieting. Now, five diets later I'm 225 pounds. I only wish I could get back to the 140 pounds where I started." It surprised me when she said, "I'm disappointed and frustrated and I don't feel like myself anymore."

What hit her hard was that she had lost weight so many times and now she was heavier than ever. The sad truth is that the majority of dieters fail to keep off the weight they lose. Most dieters not only regain the weight they initially lose but many end up with a net weight gain after dieting.[1]

The Problem with Dieting

If you've tried dieting, you've probably found out for yourself that losing weight is much easier than keeping it off. Why is this? One of the problems with diets is that they aren't sustainable. By design, diets are temporary and yield only short-term results. By the time people come to me for help to lose weight, they often tell me that they've tried many different diets, each one with the same result. Some had lost as much as one hundred pounds. In the end, they had regained all the weight they lost and more. All this to say that dieting makes things worse. Weight regain after dieting makes it important to look beyond a quick-fix diet that will likely backfire.

1

You don't have to put up with having your weight go up and down time after time. Continuous weight cycling can be prevented. I'll show you how with the book you have in your hands: *Happy Life at a Healthy Weight: Creating a Shame-Free, Healthy Relationship with Food and Life.*

Who This Book Is For

This book is dedicated to you, adults who have tried dieting to lose weight, usually repeatedly. Like Julie, you're disappointed with the results and yourself. You're fed up with dieting. You yearn for a healthy relationship with food. You feel ashamed that you lost control, slid back to overeating, and have failed to find the right solution.

I believe that you deserve to live in the sweet spot of your life, with a healthy mind and body at the weight you want to be. You deserve to live the life you've always wanted to live and look in the mirror and love who you see.

A problem in the United States is that we live in an obesogenic environment that encourages us to eat large amounts of highly processed food products filled with sugar, salt, and fat that are designed to keep us coming back for more. These foods soothe us and temporarily offer a fleeting relief from stress. At the same time, our physical environment makes it all too easy for us to become couch potatoes. We're sedentary and stationary for most of our waking hours, meaning that we burn less energy. Lastly, humans have survived over many thousands of years in part because of a strong "hunger hormone" that stimulates us to eat and that can lead to weight regain after dieting. The result? Today, almost 75 percent of Americans are overweight or obese. Many Americans suffer from diet-related health conditions, and forty of these conditions are related to obesity.

The Sweet Life Approach

My approach is to help you build a healthy relationship with food so you can live a happy life at a healthy weight. I aim to help you break free from food triggers and lifestyle choices that cause overeating. A helpful place to start is to recognize the power of healing the connection between food and shame. By transforming this connection, it is possible to free yourself from being controlled by food and stop overeating. I'll show you how. The intended result is to help you move from a place of shame and overeating to thriving.

Instead of recommending a diet, I use an empowerment model that encourages you to become an advocate and take a stand for yourself. With this book, you make the rules. You define what a healthy weight means to you. The result is a comprehensive lifestyle approach to habit change and weight loss instead of a diet. The focus is on habit changes that fit your lifestyle and that you can sustain. This comprehensive lifestyle program is designed for you to build a shame-free healthy relationship with food, lose weight, and keep it off. How it works is by removing inner roadblocks and nurturing yourself with conscious food choices, physical activity, and healthier lifestyle behaviors.

Is the Sweet Life approach relevant if you are considering weight loss approaches like surgery or medications? Yes! This comprehensive lifestyle change approach is important because the right behavior changes make the difference between weight loss success and failure. This means that without lasting lifestyle change, no other weight loss techniques, including surgery or medications, will be effective in the long run. The key to success is to consistently make better lifestyle choices that we equip you with whether or not you also choose weight loss surgery or medications.

This book takes you on a journey designed to help you discover and remove the inner and outer obstacles at play that prevent you from living a happy life at a healthy weight. I begin with the connection between food and shame, identifying the roots of shame and how it may show up in your life. Then, I show you how the cycle of overeating plays out in real life. I'll ask you to listen to and accept your feelings and embrace what you truly want. When you do that, you'll find you no longer want to eat as a way to cope with feeling empty inside or to temporarily relieve stress.

What are your other inner obstacles to losing weight and keeping it off? Let's find out. Start where you are and tackle the issues that most get in your way. Part 1 of this book helps you discover your personalized path. You'll create your Success ROADMAP to navigate your most important inner obstacles. Part 2 provides principles to help you overcome problems. Each chapter offers you a how-to guide with practical tools to easily apply relevant principles in your everyday life.

Part 3 offers you a Lifestyle Guide to put your preferred solutions into practice. This book uses a problem-focused approach that helps you avoid the trap that comes when you expect quick weight loss results and fall for a gimmicky short-term diet. Instead, I recommend that you take a stand for yourself and apply tiny habit changes that can add up and make a big difference with a comprehensive lifestyle change approach.

My Devotedly Unhealthy Relationship with Food

Back when I was eight years old, I started a devotedly unhealthy relationship with food. I experienced abuse as a child that launched me into years of hiding and shame. I began overeating to comfort myself. This turned into a habit of overeating and yo-yo dieting for years and years. Growing up in our little red house with a white picket fence, I remember that when I looked in the mirror, I didn't even like who I saw. I'll never forget that my mom loved to bake sweets and the glow of satisfaction from eating the warm, gooey chocolate chip cookies she made for me, and eating them while they were still warm, almost right out of the oven.

Eating those sweet, warm chocolate chip cookies reminded me that she loved me. This being controlled by food was an overwhelming feeling and actually compelled me to make my career choice of becoming a dietitian. I did lose 350 pounds, but not all at once. It was the same fifteen to twenty pounds that I lost repeatedly as I yo-yo dieted for decades.

Then, I met a lady who helped me see that it wasn't about what I was eating, it was about *why* I was eating, and that I had been using food to hide my shame. She showed me a process that was like a mirror reflecting the choices I was making. I used the process she showed me, and it changed my life. It wasn't until I met this lady that I solved the problem of the shame I felt from letting food control me.

Now I have a healthy relationship with food. As of fifteen years ago, I no longer overeat or yo-yo diet, and I look in the mirror and love who I see. Healthy eating (though not perfectly) became a catalyst for living the life I'd always wanted to live. What I discovered through my journey and working with hundreds of people on their nutrition, weight, and health issues is that shame and the feeling of being unworthy are at the root of most unhealthy relationships with food.

Shame happens when you don't feel safe to ask for what you deeply want at the core of who you truly are. The root cause of my shame was abuse I experienced as a child. Being controlled by food was only a symptom. Then, I turned shame into courage and stopped being controlled by food. I used the very uncomfortable feeling of shame as fuel to propel me to live the life I truly wanted to live. During this journey I stopped hiding, remembered who I truly was, and began to love who I am.

My Purpose; My Why

Now my purpose, my 'why,' is to help you break free from food triggers and heal the connection between food and shame, build a healthy relationship with food, and live a happy, sweet life at the weight you want to be. I tell you my story because I want you to know that you are not alone in having experienced difficult times in life and having used food to cope. No matter what has happened to you, I want you to know that you have a choice and can stop being controlled by food and stop using food for comfort and to hide your shame. I encourage you to take a stand and empower yourself to make changes that will allow you to triumph. The result can be for you, as it is for me, to thrive by living life with passion, purpose, compassion, and love for all who have suffered and yet summon the courage to flourish with greater health and well-being.

Kay Loughrey
December 2023

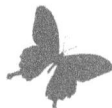

PART 1

Getting Ready for a Shame-Free, Healthy Relationship with Food

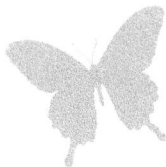

Laying the foundation about the role shame plays in your relationship with food and establishing your navigation for your weight loss journey

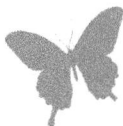

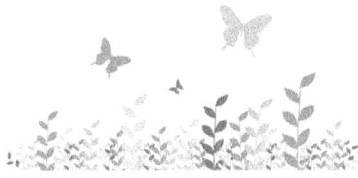

CHAPTER 1

Roots of Shame

KATIE, A WOMAN WHO CAME TO ME FOR HELP, told me that when growing up in her family, conflict wasn't allowed, and this was an unwritten family rule. As a result, there was little conversation. Katie's family conditioned her not to seek connection or conversation for fear that a family conflict might erupt.

Katie yearned to connect with other people but soon learned to keep things to herself. She hid her desire to strike up a conversation. This hiding made her feel like there was something wrong with her. Feeling that something was wrong with her engendered shame. This shame made her feel isolated and lonely because she couldn't share an important part of who she was. As a result, she felt ashamed and lonely. Then she turned to food to console and comfort herself. She came to feel that food controlled her.

This book aims to help you heal the connection between food and shame. I start by looking at the root causes of shame. Shame has three original root causes that can lead to shame and overeating:

1. Early childhood conditioning
2. Traumatic events
3. Social expectations

Katie's story is an example of childhood conditioning that began with parental conditioning that led to overeating. The second root cause of shame is trauma. In the introduction of this book, I gave you the example of trauma I experienced when I was eight years old when I felt shame, which had me repeatedly turning to food for decades to comfort myself.

Other examples of major trauma besides abuse are the death of a loved one, divorce, major illness, and combat-related Post-Traumatic Stress Disorder, typically referred to as its acronym: PTSD. Experiences like these make survivors primed to be easily triggered and go into fight, flight, or freeze responses, making them very reactive to stressful situations.

A third root cause of shame is social expectations. As a society, we have social norms about body image, as in that old saying, "you can never be too thin or too rich." Even more powerful, in many cultures, we are taught to tamp down or stuff down our feelings. Expressing our feelings is seen as a sign of weakness. So, we hide our feelings. Some ways we express this advice to tamp down our feelings are:

"Just get over it."

"Move on."

"Get a grip."

Instead, I believe our feelings can be a source of strength. When we feel worthy enough to tap into our real feelings and what we truly want, then we can summon the courage to ask for what we most want to receive. This self-awareness combined with courage can allow us to shed our shame and grow our confidence.

At a young age, we try to live up to our parents' expectations. We do what we think will bring us approval. We adjust by doing things like toning it down so we won't be a burden, dimming our light so as not to outshine a sibling, or not voicing our beliefs to avoid being criticized. Social expectations become another layer of conditioning.

Our thinking mind, known by other names such as the ego mind or inner critic, also helps to reinforce this conditioning with negative thinking and self-talk until it becomes an unconscious habit. Our ego mind often dishes out doom and gloom self-talk that tells us we'll never be successful at what we really want so why bother? This is the inner voice of shame. The ego mind's voice can be savage or seductive and it can be unrelenting if we continue to listen to it. I have found based on my personal experience and experience working with people who use food to hide their shame or feel controlled by food that the ego mind also can actively sabotage our relationship with food.

There is an alternative. Left unchecked, this connection between food and shame acts as an undercurrent in your life and as a primary inner obstacle that holds you back from building a healthy relationship with food. Your journey to free yourself from feeling controlled by food starts now. You can break the chains of hiding and shame beginning when you identify your specific connection between food and shame.

Whatever the root cause of their shame, when people first tell me their frustrations with their life, health, and weight, they say things like, "I don't feel like I'm good enough," and some even say to me, "I feel like I'm damaged goods."

Then, from that underlying shame, once triggered by a stressful event, these people often turn to food or alcohol or both for comfort or rebellion, which eventually becomes a habit.

All three root causes of shame and overeating leave a residue of shame that can cause you to hide in the shadows and deny who you truly are. Consider this: are you tired of not feeling like yourself and dissatisfied with your life and your weight? Is it time for you to take a stand for yourself and step into your strengths, so you can build a shame-free relationship with food, and live a happy life at a healthy weight? If yes, this book is meant to take you on a life-changing journey.

Chapter Summary

In this book, I aim to help you heal the connection between food and shame. The intended result is for you to move from a place of shame and overeating to thriving and flourishing. Start by looking at the root causes of shame. Shame has three original root causes that can lead to shame and overeating that is identified in this chapter. You can break the chains of hiding and shame beginning when you identify your specific connection between food and shame.

Reflection Questions

1. What's the connection between food and shame for you?

2. How do the root sources of shame show up in your life?

3. What is your food and shame story?

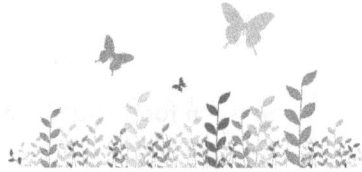

CHAPTER 2

The Food-Shame Cycle

THIS BOOK IS DEDICATED TO HELPING YOU break free from food triggers and lifestyle choices that cause overeating so you can build a healthy relationship with food. I recommend that you begin this journey by recognizing the power of healing the connection between food and shame. This chapter breaks down the five elements of the cycle of overeating. The cycle begins with an underlying shame that often comes from early childhood experiences or other roots of shame as we talked about in Chapter 1.

Stress or other emotions can trigger a fight or flight response. This response to a potential threat increases our appetite, can cause us to overeat, and perpetuates shame and stress. How does appetite come into play in the connection between food and shame? Let's look at how the brain works to explore this connection.

According to Bessel Van Der Kolk, author, researcher, and professor of psychiatry at Brown University School of Medicine, the emotional brain interferes with what we're thinking about and has a huge influence on decisions like what we choose to eat, as he described in *The Body Keeps the Score, Brain, Mind, and Body in the Healing of Trauma.*[2] The emotional brain is made up of two parts: the reptilian brain (the most primitive part of the brain in the brain stem) and the limbic system. The brainstem performs basic housekeeping functions like hunger, sleep, and breathing. The limbic system is the seat of emotions and monitors danger.

The emotional brain monitors what is dangerous and what is pleasurable. When triggered, we instantly go into Fight, Flight, Freeze, or Fawn. At the same time, our hunger increases and we then eat. In bygone eras we used that fuel to run from the saber-toothed tiger. Now we no longer need to run from the saber-toothed tiger! Today's Fight-or-Flight makes us run to the refrigerator. We Fight our shame by soothing ourselves with food. Our Flight is running to the refrigerator. Our Freeze is running to the freezer. Then we feel even more stress and more shame.

This Fight-or-Flight response easily triggers what I now label as the Food-Shame cycle, a depiction I created to illustrate how the cycle of overeating operates. It's called a cycle because it repeats itself within our brain circuitry by firing what can eventually become a default setting in response to a trigger that arises from fear and stress. Sadly, this cycle perpetuates and contributes to more stress rather than relieving it. Just what is the Food-Shame Cycle and how does it work? This cycle describes the chain of events that stimulate overeating as a way to relieve fear and stress.

The Food-Shame Cycle

Stress is most often the immediate trigger that comes from many sources; for example, a difficult conversation at work that activates an underlying root cause of shame. Once triggered, the five steps of the Food-Shame Cycle come into play. Note that it starts with shame and ends with shame, making it a vicious cycle.

1. Activated underlying shame
2. Food cravings
3. Eating for comfort
4. Feeling brief relief
5. Feelings of regret and self-disgust

The cycle repeats itself immediately or sometimes day after day.

Figure 1. Trigger and Food Shame Cycle

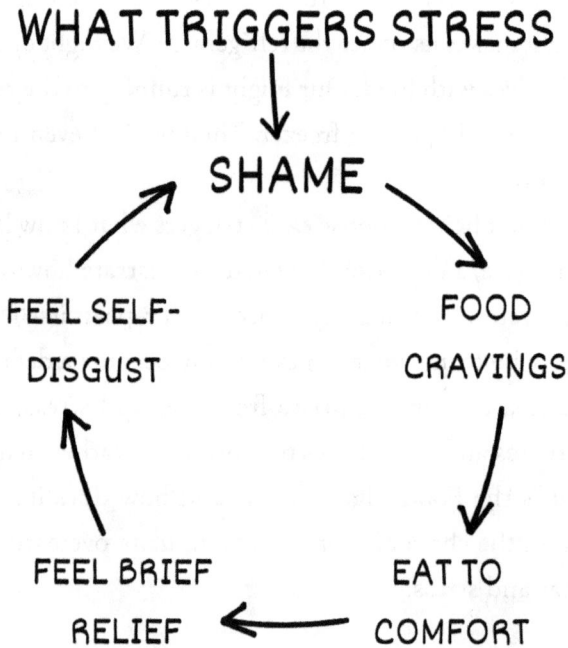

WHAT TRIGGERS STRESS

SHAME

FEEL SELF-
DISGUST

FOOD
CRAVINGS

FEEL BRIEF
RELIEF

EAT TO
COMFORT

Healing the Food-Shame Connection

What can you do to heal the vicious cycle between food and shame and stop feeling controlled by food? How long will this cycle last? I will show you how to disrupt and replace this cycle with the Five Steps to Stop Being Controlled by Food in Chapter 7. You will also receive examples of how Katie dealt with triggers and food cravings and broke the Food-Shame Cycle. Remember Katie? Katie was introduced and her source of underlying shame was described in Chapter 1.

Chapter Summary

This chapter broke down the five elements of the cycle of overeating. The cycle begins with an underlying shame that often comes from early childhood experiences or other root causes. With daily events that cause stress or other emotions, underlying shame can turn into triggers and an automatic Fight-or-Flight response accompanied by increased hunger. Then we overeat and, after brief relief, we feel more shame in the form of regret or self-disgust and greater stress. In this chapter, we described this cycle so we can then understand how this cycle of feeling controlled by food operates.

Reflection Questions

1. What daily stresses or emotions cause or trigger you to overeat?

2. What kind of food cravings do you have after being triggered and what pattern do you notice about the time of day, situation, or environment?

3. How do you feel after you eat to comfort yourself or relieve yourself from boredom or stress?

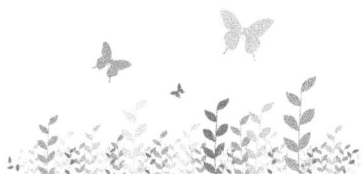

CHAPTER 3

Self-Assessment

Discover Your Inner Roadblocks

The ROADMAP is discussed in more detail later, but, as the common saying goes, "A journey of a thousand miles begins with a single step." Use the quiz below to help you identify what your most important problems you want to change on your journey toward a shame-free, healthy relationship with food will be.

Read through each of the fifteen statements below. Then, rate each statement using the following responses:

Low = This problem is of low importance to me.
Medium = This problem is of medium importance to me.
High = This problem is of high importance to me.

ROADMAP Assessment Quiz

1.	I expect quick results from diets and changing habits.	low medium high
2.	I don't make myself a priority.	low medium high
3.	I use food and alcohol as relief for mood or stress.	low medium high
4.	I don't believe I can succeed.	low medium high
5.	I am afraid to disappoint others.	low medium high
6.	I use food as a substitute for real fulfillment.	low medium high
7.	I lose track of why weight loss matters.	low medium high
8.	I apply new habits, then they fall by the wayside.	low medium high
9.	I don't know why I keep repeating old patterns.	low medium high
10.	Daily stress or lack of sleep leave me too tired for self-care.	low medium high
11.	I beat myself up or give up if I don't carry out my aims perfectly.	low medium high
12.	I forget about my body's needs. I eat quickly, while distracted, when full, or skip meals. I don't get enough sleep.	low medium high
13.	I start off strong, then I lose momentum.	low medium high
14.	I'm afraid of failing or succeeding at weight loss.	low medium high
15.	My lifestyle choices and eating are largely unconscious.	low medium high

Of those problems rated as high, what are the top three problems that you face with losing weight and keeping it off? Write down your top three problems in rank order. You'll use these three problems to find your starting point and first landmarks to your destination in the next chapter.

Chapter 4 introduces you to the ROADMAP and shows you how to navigate it to begin with the most important inner ROAD BLOCKS you face. You'll then match these problems up with principles and practical solutions in Part 2.

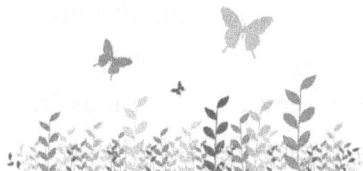

Your ROADMAP to Success

YOUR RELATIONSHIP WITH FOOD wasn't built in a day, or even a year. Events in our life can shift our relationship with food, especially traumatic events or times when we were shamed for how we looked or what we were eating. There is no one-step, one-size-fits-all solution to building a healthy relationship with food. Every situation (and every person) is unique.

Many fad diets offer a linear approach to weight loss: you eat this one food or take this one supplement and then weight loss will follow. Of course, for most people, weight gain often follows within weeks or months after finishing a temporary diet. Instead, we're seeking a comprehensive lifestyle change that lasts, and for that, we have to go beyond the one-step, linear diet plans. That's where the ROADMAP comes in.

Many of us depend on our global positioning systems (GPS) to get us where we need to go in our cars these days. While it's certainly convenient, following a GPS's directions only shows us a small portion of the larger map. If we lose a signal or there's an unexpected roadblock, we're left guessing where we should go to next. If you're lucky, or maybe just old-fashioned, you'll have a roadmap folded up somewhere in the car that will show you the entire landscape and all available routes, and maybe even some landmarks to help you along the way.

That's the approach with the ROADMAP. The fifteen problems in the ROADMAP chart below aren't designed to be solved in the order they are listed below from one to fifteen. I take a non-linear approach that shows you the lay of the land and common landmarks, and lets you remove your most important obstacles identified in your ROADMAP Quiz and follow a path best suited to you on your journey to create a shame-free, healthy relationship with food, as well as breaking the Food-Shame Cycle.

How to Use This Book

Let's partner to start your step-by-step journey to living the life you want to live at the weight you want to be. Where to begin? Start by reading Chapters 1 and 2 to discover how the connection between food and shame may be holding you back. My highest coaching recommendation is that you focus next on your top three problems, the ROADBLOCKS that most get in the way of living a happy life at a healthy weight.

I have discovered that clients do better when they focus on only one to three obstacles at any one time. Why? Changing habits takes concentration and repetition until changes are mastered. This conclusion comes from research, experience as a behavioral nutritionist and weight loss coach, and my own struggles with my weight. How? Choose and then apply the top three problems you identified from ROADMAP Assessment Quiz in Chapter 3 and use them to guide you as you use this book on your weight loss journey.

These problems each align with a chapter in Part 2: The Problems and Solutions for a Happy Life at a Healthy Weight. Pick the chapter that directly addresses your most important problem as a place to start. Then, if you want to delve further into this specific problem, pick one of the other chapters next to this problem in the chart below. Find and read the chapter that is most relevant to you. Hint: Each chapter in

Part 2 includes a Companion Chapters for Exploration section that highlights the content of related chapters as a quick way to decide which other chapters are most relevant to your needs.

You may find that a chapter you start with doesn't apply to you as much as you thought it would. That's okay. Go to another chapter and come back to any chapter as you need it. When you've finished using this book to address your top three problems, you can come back to your ROADMAP Assessment Quiz and identify your next three most important problems or go back to the table of contents and read through the chapter titles to find one that you feel will best continue your learning. There may be chapters that you read through a few times as you seek to apply them to your life and there may be chapters you never read at all. Or you can choose to read the entire book from cover to cover and then come back to the chapters that most speak to you. The greatest value of this book is to use it as a how-to guide. This book yields benefits when you apply the system of recommended behavior changes and customize them for you. Use this book however you need to—let your choices here be your first step toward changing your relationship with food!

Will you be surprised if you discover some things about yourself that you haven't thought of before? Could you be a people-pleaser and not even realize it? That's what I found out about myself as I began to look at my patterns. It's all good. That's why I suggest you approach this book with curiosity and open your heart and mind to discoveries that pave the way to living a happy life at a healthy weight.

The ROADMAP

If you identified this problem...	Read these chapters:
I expect quick results from diets and changing habits.	5: Also 8, 12, 13, 17, 19
I don't make myself a priority.	6: Also 8, 9, 11, 15, 19
I use food and or alcohol as relief for mood or stress.	7: Also 1, 2, 8, 10, 13
I don't believe I can succeed.	8: Also 6, 9, 11, 15, 18
I am afraid to disappoint others.	9: Also 6, 7, 8, 15,16
I use food as a substitute for real fulfillment.	10: Also 6, 7, 11, 13, 17
I lose track of why weight loss matters.	11: Also 8, 10, 14, 17, 18
I apply new habits, then they fall by the wayside.	12: Also 7, 8, 11, 17, 18
I don't know why I keep repeating old patterns.	13: Also 7, 8, 9, 18, 19
Daily stress or lack of sleep leave me too tired for self-care.	14: Also 5, 6, 9, 12, 16
I beat myself up or give up if I don't carry out my aims perfectly.	15: Also 7, 9, 13, 16, 19
I forget about my body's needs. I eat quickly, while distracted, when full, or skip meals. I don't get enough sleep.	16: Also 5, 6, 7, 14, 19
I start off strong, then I lose momentum.	17: Also 5, 11, 12
I'm afraid of failing or succeeding at weight loss.	18: Also 1, 7, 8, 13, 19
My lifestyle choices and eating are largely unconscious.	19: Also 7, 9, 12, 13, 18

PART 2

The Problems and Solutions for a Happy Life at a Healthy Weight

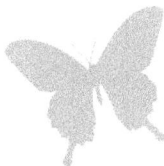

Problem-focused, solution-centered, practical ways to navigate your Success ROADMAP to a shame-free, healthy relationship with food

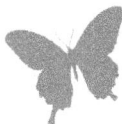

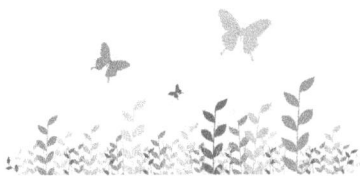

CHAPTER 5

Expectations

PROBLEM: I'm disappointed with quick fix diets and weight regain. I expect rapid results that don't last and set me further back.

PRINCIPLE: Get started. Keep going. It takes time for tiny habit changes to make a big difference. Align expectations and actions.

WHAT DOES IT MEAN TO MAKE TINY CHANGES, and how do they make a difference? When Janet first called me, she told me she wanted to lose forty pounds so she could feel better, have more energy and confidence, and be in better shape. She wanted to see her grandchildren grow up and see what they would become and what their future holds. She didn't have a lot of confidence that she could lose weight and she was afraid to fail. She had an unhelpful pattern of skipping breakfast, and sometimes she skipped lunch too, eating her first meal at dinner. Then she might grab ice cream and eat it late at night. She knew she was an emotional eater. She also had pre-diabetes.

From our partnership together, Janet made a series of tiny changes. She began by using an app to record her food intake and became much more aware of what she was eating. Then she started eating a small breakfast as a second tiny habit change. Her confidence grew as she successfully added other tiny changes over the months. She ate a small lunch each day, reined in her emotional eating, and took a three-mile walk with her husband Steve on most days. Janet and Steve had become accountability partners for each other along the way. These tiny changes added up to greater confidence, and that compounded over the months. Janet created a healthier eating pattern, is in better shape, and she's lost forty pounds, having reached her intended goal weight. She continues these tiny changes to this day with a new confidence and a belief in her ability to lose this weight and keep it off one tiny action at a time.

In fact, Steve and Janet both worked with me at the same time and each lost forty pounds by making consistent tiny changes. They reached their intended weight loss goal in nine months and are now working on maintaining their weight. They have each lost an average of a pound a week without going hungry or becoming grumpy. They are highly satisfied with their results.

Expecting Quick Weight Loss Results?

How many times have you chosen a quick-fix diet to lose weight only to see it backfire after you gave up on it because it wasn't sustainable? Lack of sustainability is at the heart of why dieting makes things worse.

Women's magazines are filled with weight-loss tips during the summer. Recently, my eyes scanned the cover of an issue as I stood in a grocery line. I read the headline, "Lose 36 Pounds by Memorial Day" with rapt attention. Is it possible to lose this much weight in a few weeks? The short answer is that this outcome is extremely rare. To my surprise, Candice, a woman I'm working with, lost twenty-four pounds in the first four weeks of her weight loss journey after she stopped drinking a whopping eight sodas a day! Candice's experience with this amount of rapid weight loss is unusual among the many adults I have helped lose weight in the last twelve years. She had changed just one bad habit with a profound effect.

Most adults who I help lose an average of one to two pounds a week by making a combination of tiny changes that compound over time with small, consistent actions.

Outlandish promises may give us a momentary thrill, and yet diets that promise quick results with little effort usually create outsized expectations followed by crushing disappointment. Many of us fall for weight loss promises that are too good to be true, just like many people fall for those fake get-rich-quick schemes that are just as alluring. These gimmicks can lead us to expect that we are just one magic trick away from melting off fat and extra pounds—that come off quickly and stay off forever without any real effort.

For me, I lost the same fifteen to twenty pounds more than twenty-five times as a yo-yo dieter until I stopped dieting and lost weight in a sustainable way. Dieting had become an obsession to distract me as I hid from other challenges in my life that I didn't want to face. I swung from feast to famine and back again. I spent days feasting on extra sweets as I got ready for a diet—the famine. I felt guilty and ashamed after cheating on diets, while at the same time, I looked forward to all the chocolate treats I would eat after the diet ended.

Most people who have tried dieting feel good at first about their initial weight loss success. Sadly, these results aren't usually lasting. Dieters who lose weight usually regain 80 percent of the weight they lost within five years.[3]

Let's look at Sandy, a woman I met at a health fair. She told me the story of how she'd lost fifty pounds on a popular diet. Then, she stopped the diet because she couldn't afford to continue buying the company's food. The result was that she regained the fifty pounds she initially lost, plus she gained another twenty pounds. When people first come to me, they often tell me that they've tried many different diets with initial success and the same disappointing result in the long run. Yet, a real weight loss solution without dieting is available to you, in contrast to continuing with guilt and shame associated with yo-yo dieting and weight cycling.

What Gets in the Way

Many of us are looking for the right solution to help us lose the extra weight we carry. On average, we Americans in the US gained twenty or more pounds during the pandemic and still struggle to lose this excess weight.4 COVID-19 aside, our environment causes us to easily gain extra weight. There's even a special term for what causes us to gain weight—our obesogenic (obesity-inducing) environment. Three aspects of our environment contribute to weight gain:

1. OUR FOOD SUPPLY

We Americans have an abundant supply of processed and ultra-processed food that makes us gain weight and damages our mental and physical health.[5] Since the 60s Americans have increased the average BMI from twenty-five to twenty-eight in the year 2002. This increase in BMI is in direct correlation of Americans having plentiful access to cheap, convenient foods so that by now almost 75 percent of US adults carry extra weight and are considered overweight or obese.[6]

Why was this happening? The food industry with $8.33 trillion in sales in 2023, churns out more and more cheap, super-sized processed food products filled with salt, sugar, and saturated fat. As a result, people have been getting sicker and sicker because of skyrocketing rates of diabetes and obesity. I was shocked by how much the number of people diagnosed with diabetes grew over the years: from 1.6 million Americans diagnosed with diabetes in 1958 to 23.4 million diagnosed in 2015. That is an astronomical 1,463 percent increase in Americans diagnosed with diabetes in fifty-seven years![7]

2. SEDENTARY LIFESTYLE

We live sedentary lives. Most of our time is spent nearly motionless in front of devices like smartphones and computer screens whether we are at work or play. The result is that we burn a fraction of the energy required by our physically active hunter-gather and farmer ancestors.

3. CHRONIC STRESS

Many of us also live stress-filled lives in a state of chronic stress, which leaves us feeling that our lives are out of control. And yet, something is missing. We may feel controlled by the sheer pace of life and use food, alcohol, or other drugs to numb our feelings. We try to relieve ourselves of chronic stress and feelings of emptiness with food and alcohol as relief for our mood and stress.

Tiny Changes that Make a Big Difference

Maybe you yearn to make sweeping changes and create a whole new healthy eating pattern and lifestyle. I'm here to tell you that taking on massive lifestyle changes all at once is much harder to sustain and can be overwhelming. It's much more effective to systematically make tiny changes with individual, targeted behaviors practiced consistently over time. This combination is designed to help you build confidence, consistency, and sustainable behaviors. That's how you can get on a roll with the momentum needed to go the distance and make a big difference.

Real change takes patience, persistence, and perseverance. Patience suggests steadfastness. While the dictionary definition of persistence suggests continued effort despite obstacles, perseverance takes action further. With perseverance, effort continues despite difficulties or opposition that exceeds the usual obstacles that may include inertia or lack of self-confidence. With any change there is a learning curve that starts with a process that moves you through a try-out period—often with lots of mistakes, plus skill building, competence, and finally with creating a new normal. In this book, I show you how to make tiny changes consistently to master habit changes, go the distance, and make a big difference in your quality of life.

By my mid-twenties, when I was studying for a degree in nutrition and dietetics, I realized that dieting made things worse and kept me in a continuous tailspin with my weight constantly fluctuating up and down. The more I dieted, the worse things got. Then I discovered an alternative: the idea of habit change. I was delighted to find a little book in the 1980s, *Habits Not Diets: The Secret to Lifetime Weight Control* by James M. Ferguson, which illuminated an alternative to dieting about how to use self-observation and a small steps approach to achieve and maintain weight loss.[8] I've used a habit approach since that time for myself and the people I help. The result has been that I eat my favorite sweet treats consciously and selectively as I decide how much and how often to enjoy them without guilt or shame. I also continue to study developments on habit change theory and practice.

How many food and lifestyle choices do you make in a day, like what to eat and when to go to bed? From working with people like Janet and Steve, it's become evident that the tiny choices you make every day can take you either toward or away from the life you want to live. I am lucky because a few years ago one of my business mentors, Jamey Schrier, gave me a book that made a tremendous difference in my understanding of how consistent actions can bring success and inaction can bring dismal failure. Darren Hardy, former publisher of *Success Magazine* and author of *The Compound Effect, Multiplying Your Success One Simple Step at a Time*, explained that consistency is the key to success.[9] He showed how these simple steps compound over time to yield a huge payoff from consistently making the right small choices and turning them into small steps.

More recently, I studied James Clear's book, *Atomic Habits: An Easy and Proven Way to Build Good Habits and Break Bad Ones*, another habit change resource that added new insights to habit change and clearly explained the impact of making tiny changes.[10] He wrote that tiny changes or 1 percent improvements, can make an astounding difference in the long run. In other words, what you do each day accumulates. Clear explained that by making one tiny improvement each day builds to a thirty-seven-times better outcome over a year. And a 1 percent improvement not only sounds doable, but sustainable and practical. The opposite is also true. Tiny mistakes or inaction also accumulate into a gradual decline that eventually can become a serious problem. His recommendation was to create not just changes, but a system of 1 percent changes to achieve a desired outcome.

Chapter Summary

In this chapter, you were introduced to the fallacy of expecting rapid and lasting results with a quick fix diet that is temporary. Instead, you have been guided to use a comprehensive lifestyle approach that emphasizes making tiny changes that can make a big difference because they can be sustained for a lifetime (though not perfectly). These changes require patience, persistence, and perseverance to create a shame-free healthy relationship with food for a happy life at a healthy weight

Companion Chapters for Exploration

Want more help with the problem that you expect quick results that ultimately sets you back? Here's a recommended shortcut: pick one or more of the chapters below to read next that seem most relevant to you. (These are also listed on the ROADMAP chart in Chapter 4.)

MINDSET: I DON'T BELIEVE I CAN SUCCEED (CHAPTER 8)

Explore how your mindset and beliefs from the past may interfere with weight loss and how to cultivate a mindset shift that will help you master new habits.

LACK OF CONSISTENCY: NEW HABITS FALL BY THE WAYSIDE (CHAPTER 12)

Changing habits consistently is the Golden Key to solving the problem posed in this chapter: "I Apply New Habits, Then They Fall by the Wayside." This chapter demonstrates how to build new habits with consistency and sustain new habits.

FEELING STUCK: I KEEP REPEATING OLD PATTERNS (CHAPTER 13)

It's far easier to repeat old patterns when we aren't present in the moment and are unconscious of the choices we are making. In this chapter, I share how to heal the past, embrace the present, and choose your future.

INSPIRING ACTION: I START OUT STRONG, THEN I LOSE MOMENTUM (CHAPTER 17)

This chapter is built on the question, "How can you keep up your momentum once you discover your top motivators for a happy life at a healthy weight?" In this chapter, I share a big secret to weight loss success is inspired daily commitment called recommitment.

TUNED OUT: MY LIFESTYLE CHOICES ARE LARGELY UNCONSCIOUS (CHAPTER 19)

For many of us, lifestyle choices are largely unconscious, and that causes us to overeat and forget about self-care. I share essential advantages and aspects of making conscious choices, including paying attention while eating and slowing down enough so you can tell when you're full without overeating.

Reflection Questions

Begin your journey now to a shame-free healthy relationship with food so you can live a happy life at a healthy weight by confirming whether our comprehensive lifestyle change approach is right for you.

Place a check on statements below that resonate with you:

☐ Past dieting has worked only temporarily for me. Eventually, I go back to old habits.

☐ I want a solution that gets to the root cause of my weight issues instead of just dealing with outer symptoms so I can live the life I want to live at a healthy weight.

☐ I see that my extra weight stems from inner triggers and I want to stop soothing myself with food.

☐ I am looking for a solution that will help me build a shame-free, healthy relationship with food so I can make better food choices and have a lifestyle I can sustain.

☐ I appreciate the idea of finding a comprehensive lifestyle change approach that will help me build good habits, lose weight, and keep it off once and for all. I don't want to invest my time and money over and over again on a quick-fix diet.

I invite you to take the journey and discover your path to a happy life at a healthy weight by following the plan outlined in this book if these five key elements resonate with you.

How-To Guide

QUICK LIFE HACK

Identify the first tiny change you want to make in what, when, where, or how you will eat this week to get started on your path to a healthy relationship with food.

Example: I plan to make better choices when I eat out this week by either skipping the bread, alcoholic or sweet beverages, or dessert or ordering an appetizer instead of a main course.

GUIDEBOOK EXERCISES

Exercise 1: Create Your Path

Exercise 2: Set Yourself Up for Success

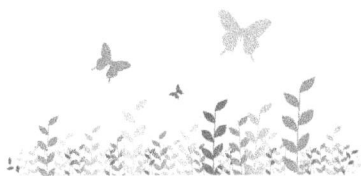

CHAPTER 6

Running on Empty

PROBLEM: I don't make myself a priority.

PRINCIPLE: Declare your worthiness and make yourself a priority.

MAKING YOURSELF A PRIORITY is the top guiding core principle for the Sweet Life Wellness weight loss plan. This principle is the mother of all other core principles, because with it, we can overcome all other obstacles to having a fulfilling life at a healthy weight. Without making yourself a priority, none of the core principles matter. If you do what's important, where do you fit in your daily priorities? Do you believe you are worthy of devoting time to your self-care? This kind of self-care makes your body and mind thrive like a car that runs with a fully charged battery and fully fueled instead of running on empty.

How Jenny Made Herself a Priority

During our first call together, Jenny mentioned that she was frustrated with constantly thinking about food and felt anxious, almost hopeless about her lack of control over her eating, weight gain, and negative mood. She had food cravings and needed help. She said she had lost weight before and was able to keep it off for almost two years. Challenges around work and parents were a source of stress that caused her to think about food all the time. Her overeating occurred mostly at home after work. She didn't think she was eating the right food since she got hungry in the afternoon and when she got home from work. She believed she needed to figure out how to eat the right foods beforehand so she could quit eating while she cooked dinner. Jenny had a highly responsible job, a daily commute, and was part of a sandwich generation, caring for both her children and ailing parents who were looking to her for help.

What Jenny really wanted was to feel like food wasn't controlling her. She also wanted to be a good role model for her daughter. Her goal was to lose twenty-five pounds and feel good, have more energy, and look better because she fit into the clothes she wanted to wear. Her vision of success was to have better mental health and not be preoccupied with food. She yearned to feel more positive and have a greater peace of mind. We did an assessment and discovered techniques that helped her make self-care a priority so she could manage stress and emotional eating. Exactly how did Jenny accomplish this feat? One technique that helped was to disrupt the pattern of stress and eating once she got home. Based on our work together, when she walked in the door, she immediately switched gears. She walked to her bedroom, showered, changed clothes, and did a ten-minute relaxation exercise. When she began to cook dinner, she was more relaxed and less likely to eat while cooking. She was happy with her results because, as she said, she now had a healthy relationship with food and it didn't control her anymore.

Are You Worth Making Yourself a Priority?

My Story: I hid and felt unworthy when I began a devotedly unhealthy relationship with food, which started when I was eight years old. I had experienced abuse that caused me to comfort myself with food, overeat for years, and yo-yo diet for decades. When I looked in the mirror, I didn't even like who I saw. Fortunately, I turned my life around, as I shared in the introduction of this book. You, too, can summon your courage and use the food-shame connection you have likely felt to transform your life, make yourself a priority, and have a shame-free healthy relationship with food and a happy life at a healthy weight.

Is Self-Care Selfish?

Sometimes we might feel unworthy because of events or even trauma from our past. The social expectation that reminds us to focus on others instead of ourselves can make it seem like self-care is selfish. We can sometimes get so wrapped up in other people and what they think that we forget to take care of ourselves. Let's delve into the popular social idea that self-care is selfish and that it's better to give than receive. Is it true? Won't you and the people around you be better off when you are in a better mood, more engaged and productive, and not just surviving? The idea of giving from an empty cup often makes for resentment.

Recall the instructions that flight attendants give before takeoff. They tell you that in case of loss of cabin pressure put your oxygen mask on first, and then help others. Why is that? Because you need oxygen to stay conscious and perform this life-saving maneuver for others. As Vietnamese Zen Master Thich Nhat Han wrote in his booklet *How to Love,* "Until you are able to love and take care of yourself, you can't be of much help to others."[11]

This notion that self-care is selfish is becoming less popular as people begin to discover that burnout is fruitless as a way of life, and they no longer want to pursue giving every fiber of their being to work as a way of life.

Josie, a young woman in her twenties, came to me for help with her weight. Her life revolved around her work as a manager. She told me that she skipped breakfast and lunch and ate mostly in the evening. While at work during the day, she ate a bite of a croissant and had a small spoonful of gelato. By the time she met with her boss at 5:00 p.m., she couldn't think clearly. She had brain fog and she wasn't able to concentrate. Her boss noticed her lack of concentration and said, "You really need to eat more regularly so you have the energy to keep going."

We collaborated on ways she could make self-care work for her. I suggested that she prepare and eat a small breakfast at home, and pack lunch, and fill a bottle of water to take with her to work. Josie decided to make these her goals for the week and it made a huge difference in how well she functioned at work. A week later she shared, "You know what? Now I see how I'm able to advocate for myself."

She no longer viewed her healthier eating pattern through the lens of lack and restriction. As a result, she had the energy and the stamina for her workouts, she lost weight and was stronger. Josie is an example of what's possible when we transform our habits and make ourselves a priority.

I have come to understand that making yourself a priority isn't just a good idea, but it also makes all the difference in your health, well-being, and weight. The focus in this book is to empower you by making yourself a priority.

Chapter Summary

This chapter revealed what it takes to commit to daily self-care, cultivate a belief that you are worthy, and adopt a belief that self-care is not selfish. The next sections are designed for you to further apply how to make yourself a priority so you can have a happy life at a healthy weight.

Companion Chapters for Exploration

Want more help with the problem that you don't make yourself a priority? Here's a recommended shortcut: pick one or more of the chapters below to read next that seem most relevant to you. (These are also listed on the ROADMAP chart in Chapter 4.)

MINDSET: I DON'T BELIEVE I CAN SUCCEED (CHAPTER 8)

We explore how your mindset and beliefs from the past may interfere with weight loss, and how to cultivate a mindset shift that will help you master new habits.

PEOPLE-PLEASING: I'M AFRAID TO DISAPPOINT OTHERS (CHAPTER 9)

People-pleasing causes us to trim our sails in life about what's possible because we are worried about what other people think and with winning their acceptance and approval instead of scheduling time for self-care. This chapter addresses what you can do about people-pleasing and what other people think.

MOTIVATION: I LOSE TRACK OF WHY WEIGHT LOSS MATTERS (CHAPTER 11)

In this chapter, we emphasize how easy it is to lose sight of your why—that is, why weight loss matters. Instead, we give you helpful ways to get and stay motivated during your weight loss journey. We also show you how to keep your reasons to lose weight in full sight. We ask you to envision the kind of person you want to become and change conflicting beliefs that can help you stay focused during your weight loss journey.

PERFECTIONISM HOLDS ME BACK: I BEAT MYSELF UP OR GIVE UP IF I DON'T CARRY OUT MY AIMS PERFECTLY (CHAPTER 15)

Judging yourself and beating yourself up are symptoms of perfectionism and cause you to give up on cherished dreams. Curiosity, compassion, and self-acceptance can allow us to make progress instead of being paralyzed by fear of being a failure when we don't carry out our aims flawlessly.

TUNED OUT: MY LIFESTYLE CHOICES ARE LARGELY UNCONSCIOUS (CHAPTER 19)

For many of us, lifestyle choices are largely unconscious, and that causes us to overeat and forget about self-care. We share essential advantages and aspects of making conscious choices, including paying attention while we eat and slowing down enough so we can tell when we're full without overeating.

Reflection Questions

It takes awareness and persistence to have a fulfilling life at a healthy weight. What about you? Reflect on your own experience with making yourself a priority by answering these questions:

1. How does not making self-care a priority show up in your life?

2. What is an example of a time when you felt guilty for taking time for self-care from the belief that self-care is selfish? What could you do differently next time?

3. What would have to happen to make yourself and self-care a priority? What will you commit to doing?

How-To Guide

QUICK LIFE HACK

Pick one action you'll take to begin making yourself a priority. For example, pack your lunch the night before if you usually skip lunch or don't have the foods available that will support you with weight loss.

GUIDEBOOK EXERCISE

Exercise 3: Finding the Time

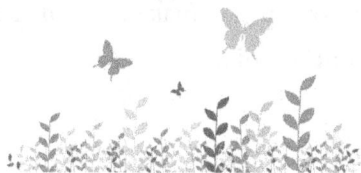

CHAPTER 7

Self-Soothing

PROBLEM: I use food/alcohol as relief for mood or stress.

PRINCIPLE: Tune into cravings and the emotions connected with them. Tap into true wishes and make better choices.

REMEMBER KATIE, FROM CHAPTER 1?[12] When she was a child, she discovered that in her family, conflict wasn't allowed—it was an unwritten family rule. Her family conditioned her not to seek connection or conversation. In a moment, you'll see that now, adult Katie has just yet again cooked a family meal for her kids and husband after a long workday and commute. When dinner is finished, no one even says thank you and they just get up and leave the table. This experience with her family each night triggered her feelings of underlying shame from childhood. Her childhood shame came from feeling that there was something wrong with her because she yearned to connect with others.

She wants to connect with her family at dinner, but instead they eat in silence and leave the table without making any real effort to interact with her. What set things off for Katie? We'll soon look at how this cycle played out before and after she applied the five steps after we cover the fundamentals of this five-step process.

Many of the clients I work with say, "I don't feel like I'm good enough," and some have even said to me, "I feel like I'm damaged goods."

Once triggered by a stressful event, these adults turn to food or alcohol or both for comfort or rebellion, which eventually becomes a habit. As an example, when Katie first called me for help, she said, "I get angry, sad, and lonely and I stuff my face. Then I feel ashamed."

After bouts of overeating intended to comfort themselves, clients I've worked with tell me that at first, they feel relieved, but then they often feel even worse. They feel a mood boost for a moment, then feel more stress and guilt. Next, they may eat even more out of self-disgust, saying to themselves, "I've already eaten five donuts, I may as well eat a few more."

These individuals have told me that the result of this cycle was that they felt controlled by food and got caught up in the vicious Food-Shame Cycle that I introduced in Chapter 2.

According to Judson Brewer, Associate Professor of Medicine and Psychiatry at the University of Massachusetts Medical School, "We have conditioned ourselves to deal with stress in ways that ultimately perpetuate it rather than release us from it."[13]

What we think helps our stress and shame only makes it worse. That's why this Food-Shame pattern becomes a vicious cycle.

When working with clients like Katie, I help them recognize and break the Food-Shame Cycle. I created these five steps to help people immediately let go of their shame and related feelings so they can break free of the Food-Shame Cycle.

Five Steps to Stop Being Controlled by Food:

Step 1: What's Your Trigger?

What's the trigger, what sets off your food cravings?

The stress trigger could be as simple as walking in the door and then into the pantry after a stressful day or being yelled at by the boss.

Once you've identified the trigger, write it down in the worksheet below.

STEP 2: WHAT'S YOUR CRAVING?

What specific food are you craving? Write it down. Maybe it's ice cream or potato chips, foods high in salt, fat, and/or sugar designed to stir up food cravings so you'll keep eating.

The problem is that these are processed, industrialized foods that only lead to more shame after we've eaten them. But here's the thing: processed food is not going to help you process shame.

STEP 3: PAUSE AND SLOW DOWN FOR A MINUTE

When triggered, pause and slow down instead of going into automatic pilot. Stop and pause. Notice the seductive ego voice that reinforces a conditioned response and continued shame by urging unwanted behaviors with, "I deserve this. I've worked hard. It's time for a reward."

STEP 4: CHECK IN WITH YOURSELF

This is the most important step in the five-step process. Now, ask yourself: "What am I feeling right now? What is it that I really want?"

Write these two things down.

What you're yearning for usually isn't food. Unless you really *are* hungry.

STEP 5: WHAT ARE YOUR CHOICES?

How can you positively respond to your cravings, emotions, and what you really want without eating?

Create a few options that are easy to remember. Then, pick the best option. Write them down and keep them handy. Be ready for the next food craving.

Here's how Katie applied the Five Steps to Stop Being Controlled by Food:

STEP 1: KATIE'S TRIGGER

Katie's trigger started right after dinner when her kids and husband silently went their own ways, and she was left alone. She turned on the TV.

STEP 2: KATIE'S CRAVING

Katie's first craving started after being triggered and then she turned on the TV. This craving caused her to reach for her favorite beer.

STEP 3: TIME TO PAUSE

Before she learned the five steps, Katie gave herself an excuse with that conditioned seductive voice of shame that said, "I deserve this reward. It's been a long, hard day, and I just fixed dinner." After learning the five steps, she paused, slowed down, and took a few slow, deep breaths to relax.

STEP 4: KATIE CHECKS IN WITH HERSELF

Before, Katie had played out the Food-Shame Cycle every weeknight. Her automatic response led to an evening of emotional eating and drinking where she felt relief for the first few minutes after drinking beer. Then she felt self-disgust and continued to drink and eat. She repeated the Food-Shame Cycle throughout the evening.

Once she learned the five steps, Katie checked in with herself. She knew she was angry because her family had ignored her and she felt lonely. Let's look at Katie's choices and what she did about her loneliness in Step 5:

- ❖ Before, Katie used to fight her shame, indulge her cravings, and soothe herself by drinking three or four strong beers and eating a bag of chips and a bowl of ice cream every weeknight. Afterwards, she felt angry, ashamed, and lonely.

- ❖ Using the five steps, Katie chose to connect with someone— something that she yearned for as her cure for loneliness instead of turning to eating for relief—a relief that made her feel better only for a few minutes. Her options were to:
  - ♦ Go for a walk with the neighbors
  - ♦ Call her sister
  - ♦ Talk with her daughter

Katie decided that her best option was to call her sister. With practice, Katie turned her reaction to a stress trigger that had activated her underlying shame into a positive response to her yearnings. This is how she broke free from the vicious Food-Shame Cycle.

LET'S LOOK AT WHAT HAD JUST HAPPENED FOR KATIE:

The shame kicked in when Katie's family members got up and left her, which triggered her underlying shame from childhood. She recognized that shame from childhood that was at the base of her response. Yet, Katie successfully dealt with the triggers and food cravings and broke the cycle. Her big Aha Moment was when she realized, "I don't have to process the underlying shame each time. I just need to recognize what is happening, recognize I've been triggered, and break the cycle using the five simple steps."

Chapter Summary

This chapter revealed that the ways we try to deal with stress may actually make it worse. This may cause us to overeat and feel controlled by food. I shared the Five Steps to Stop Being Controlled by Food and an example of how Katie dealt with triggers and food cravings and broke the Food-Shame Cycle. Remember, the next time you walk into your kitchen and open the cupboard, you don't need to open triggers, hide, and feel shame. You don't need to play a game of hide and seek with your life anymore. Instead, you can open the true you and do it with freedom and joy.

Companion Chapters for Exploration

Want more help with the problem that you use food and or alcohol as relief for mood or stress? Here's a recommended shortcut: pick one or more of the chapters below to read next that seem most relevant to you. (These are also listed on the ROADMAP chart in Chapter 4.)

ROOTS OF SHAME (CHAPTER 1)

This chapter addresses the fear of letting go of childhood survival mechanisms that once served us well but can become underlying shame that leads to overeating.

FOOD-SHAME CYCLE (CHAPTER 2)

In this chapter, I break down the five elements of the cycle of overeating. The cycle begins with an underlying shame that often comes from early childhood experiences. This shame turns into triggers and an automatic fight or flight response along with overeating, which perpetuates shame and stress.

MINDSET: I DON'T BELIEVE I CAN SUCCEED (CHAPTER 8)

Explores how your mindset and beliefs from the past may interfere with weight loss and how to cultivate a mindset shift that will help you master new habits.

EMPTINESS: I USE FOOD AS A SUBSTITUTE FOR REAL FULFILLMENT (CHAPTER 10)

This chapter examines how ignoring what you truly long for can lead to overeating as a cheap substitute for living the life you've always wanted to live and how you can be guided by what you truly yearn for.

FEELING STUCK: I KEEP REPEATING OLD PATTERNS (CHAPTER 13)

It's far easier to repeat old patterns when we aren't present in the moment and are unconscious of the choices we are making. This chapter shares how to heal the past, embrace the present, and choose your future.

Reflection Questions

Being aware of the food-shame connection and these five steps isn't enough. You need to recognize the food-shame connection for yourself. Use the questions below. Take a few minutes to write down your answers:

1. What situations tend to cause you to overeat?

2. What shame might you be pushing down?

How-To Guide

QUICK LIFE HACK

Note and write down:

> ✧ What situations trigger your food cravings?
>
> ✧ What feelings bring on your food cravings?

When you feel a food craving start, ride out the craving with your breath. Inhale and acknowledge the craving. Then release the craving as you exhale (repeat this breathing exercise until the craving subsides).

GUIDEBOOK EXERCISES

Exercise 4: Five Steps to Stop Being Controlled by Food Worksheet
Exercise 5: Stress Response

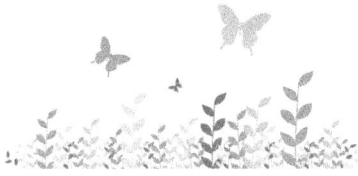

CHAPTER 8

Mindset

PROBLEM: I don't believe I can succeed at weight loss.

PRINCIPLE: Change your mindset, change your life.

JEANETTE, WHO WAS JUST ABOUT TO TURN SIXTY, called me because she wanted to lose weight. She told me that she wanted to become a good example of healthy aging. She had thought it through and knew she wanted to become fit and healthy as she continued to become older. She was a tutor who gave her life to helping her students. She had big challenges because of her busy schedule and long work hours. On weekdays, she ate dinner in the car at stop lights in the evening while driving between one client and another. She found herself writing emails at 1:30 a.m. to keep up the pace. She also volunteered for several organizations.

Jeanette knew she wanted help with eating and making time to be more physically active. But how? The first thing we did was an assessment about what was getting in the way of her desire to lose weight. Besides her dedication to her students and her busy schedule, Jeanette had one important thing going for her and that was her mindset about who she wanted to be. And, she was determined and an action taker.

Jeanette's work-life balance was another matter. She had dedicated her life to helping her students without regard to her need for self-care. We helped Jeanette change her mindset about her long work hours that were a major ROADBLOCK to her intention to become fit and healthy and lose weight. From her assessment, I recommended a series of small changes. Although it wasn't easy, Jeanette decided to shift her work life balance because of a clear vision to become an example of healthy aging. Her priorities had shifted. With the right mindset, she began to give herself time back. She scheduled a specific time to end her work day. Then she created an auto-reply email to our clients that said, "If your email is sent in after 5:00 p.m., it will be answered the next business day." And she scheduled a regular bedtime. She made many changes that gave her more energy and more time to fit in her morning workouts. She was stronger and satisfied with her quality of life. She also became an inspiration to her daughters of what healthy aging could look like.

What is your desired future? What is getting in your way, including what you are telling yourself about your ability to lose weight? This chapter explores how your mindset and beliefs from the past may interfere with weight loss, and how to cultivate a mindset shift that will help you master new habits. Mindset is fundamental for your weight loss success because you put the brakes on your progress with an inner ROADBLOCK when you believe you're going to fail before you even start your weight loss journey. I believe you deserve to have a fulfilling life, one that includes a healthy mind and a healthy body at the weight you want to be, and the ability to look in the mirror and love who you see. Otherwise, you wouldn't be reading this book. To get there, you'll need to become aware of and remove beliefs that are inner ROADBLOCKs.

Mindset is important because if we have beliefs that interfere with what we really want, it's easy to sabotage ourselves. So, let's look at what mindset means. Mindset usually shows up as self-talk that represents an attitude and a set of beliefs about a particular skill. In terms of mindset, beliefs are everything. Beliefs are powerful and that's why whether you think you can or think you can't, you're right. You get to choose. If your mindset seems fixed and you want a change, you can start migrating a specific belief towards a growth mindset. Here's how: show some flexibility, try out new things, and see what works. Can you give yourself some grace and believe it's possible to build new beliefs and habits?

My Limited Mindset

Here's my real-life example of a time when I didn't believe in myself. In high school, a "Breakfast of Champions" speaker at a school assembly sparked a dream in me to inspire people to a better life. Then I said to myself, "No one's going to listen to you. You're not a speaker or athlete, you're just a young flabby girl, and you're not even famous." And that's how I abandoned my dream as an adolescent to become a motivational speaker.

Much later, as a nutritionist and dietitian, I saw that people were getting sicker and sicker. I knew I had to do something. I had an important message to get across, because people were getting sick from their extra weight. A speaker coach showed me how to use my voice to help people live a better life and build a shame free, healthy relationship with food for a happy life and healthy weight.

What does my story from high school have to do with mindset? I had cast away a dream for myself as impossible because of my limited mindset. I didn't believe in myself. Then, six years ago, I summoned the courage to pursue my desire to be a transformational speaker and began working with a speaker coach. I realized that my calling was to share an important message, which included speaking to groups about how to build a healthy relationship with food and ways to stop sabotaging themselves with old beliefs that their dreams and wishes are impossible.

A Deeper Dive into Mindset

Which sounds more like you? Do you believe that intelligence can be acquired, or that it is something you are born with and is innate? It turns out that how people view their intelligence predicts how willing they are to learn new things and overcome challenges. Carol Dweck wrote an enlightening book, *Mindset: The New Psychology of Success*, affirming that you can change your mindset from fixed to a growth mindset, and she showed her readers how to view learning as a welcome challenge rather than a possible failure to avoid.[14]

These are the key differences between a fixed and growth mindset: Someone with a fixed mindset about something:

- Believes in innate intelligence
- Doesn't attempt difficult tasks
- Expects to fail
- Gives up easily

This is because when you have a fixed mindset about something, you don't think you can grow. You're either good at something or you're not. You can either do something or you can't.

On the other hand, someone with a growth mindset about something:

- Believes in acquired intelligence
- Likes a good challenge
- Is curious about how to overcome difficulties

✧   Believes that trying is how you succeed

What does mindset have to do with weight management? Everything, as it turns out. People who have a fixed mindset believe that losing weight means being strong and using willpower, something that you either have or you don't. On the other hand, people with a growth mindset know that they can learn, and they apply new weight loss strategies. With a fixed mindset, people tend to make an earnest and superficial effort to lose weight and then hope for the best. Then they beat themselves up when they fail. Persons with a growth mindset make a special effort and employ effective strategies and systems to make change happen. Mindset can make a difference in whether or not a person is able to lose weight and then keep it off.

Beliefs and Attitudes that Can Hold You Back

Hidden beliefs, attitudes, and underlying assumptions can sabotage your weight loss efforts. Are any of these beliefs and attitudes keeping you from taking the next step?

✧   "It's too hard—I don't want to sacrifice and starve myself."

✧   "I'll have to exercise—I don't like physical activity."

✧   "I won't get the support I need—I'll just regain the weight I lose."

Such attitudes may include fundamental beliefs about your ability to change and learn new behaviors. Do you believe, for example, that you can learn new eating behaviors and successfully make lifestyle changes that will lead you to a healthy weight?

Chapter Summary

This chapter has explored how your mindset and beliefs from the past may interfere with weight loss, and how to cultivate a mindset shift that will help you master new habits. The first step is to become aware of your mindset and discover what beliefs hamper your ability to lose weight.

Companion Chapters for Exploration

Want more help with the problem that you don't believe you can succeed? Here's a recommended short cut: pick one or more of the chapters below to read next that seem most relevant to you. (These are also listed on the ROADMAP chart in Chapter 4.)

RUNNING ON EMPTY: I DON'T MAKE MYSELF A PRIORITY (CHAPTER 6)

This chapter shows how to commit daily to declaring your worthiness and making yourself a priority. You are given tips on how to make time for yourself and schedule daily self-care and recognize that self-care is not selfish.

PEOPLE-PLEASING: I'M AFRAID TO DISAPPOINT OTHERS (CHAPTER 9)

People-pleasing causes us to trim our sails in life about what's possible because we are worried about what other people think and with winning their acceptance and approval instead of scheduling time for self-care. This chapter addresses what you can do about people-pleasing and what other people think.

MOTIVATION: I LOSE TRACK OF WHY WEIGHT LOSS MATTERS (CHAPTER 11)

In this chapter, I emphasize how easy it is to lose sight of your why—that is, why weight loss matters. Instead, you are given helpful ways to get and stay motivated during your weight loss journey. You are also shown how to keep your reasons to lose weight in full sight. Then, you are asked to envision the kind of person you want to become and change conflicting beliefs that can help you stay focused during your weight loss journey.

PERFECTIONISM: I BEAT MYSELF UP OR GIVE UP IF I DON'T CARRY OUT MY AIMS PERFECTLY (CHAPTER 15)

Judging yourself and beating yourself up are symptoms of perfectionism and cause you to give up on cherished dreams. Curiosity, compassion, and self-acceptance can allow us to make progress instead of being paralyzed by fear of being a failure when we don't carry out our aims flawlessly.

BUILDING CONFIDENCE: I'M AFRAID OF FAILING OR SUCCEEDING AT WEIGHT LOSS (CHAPTER 18)

Are you afraid when you think about losing weight? This chapter focuses on how fear can easily lead to self-sabotage and sidetrack you from your intentions. Instead, it is recommended that you focus on the things you can change as you make lifestyle choices that will support you on your weight loss journey. Then you are offered ways to choose your future with a change process and ways you can choose your response to events for a better outcome.

TUNED OUT: MY LIFESTYLE CHOICES ARE LARGELY UNCONSCIOUS (CHAPTER 19)

For many of us, lifestyle choices are largely unconscious, and that causes us to overeat and forget about self-care. In this chapter, you receive essential advantages and aspects of making conscious choices, including paying attention while eating and slowing down enough to determine cues of feeling full without overeating.

Reflection Questions

1. What is my mindset about weight loss? What do I believe is possible?

2. Can I learn new eating behaviors and lifestyle changes that will lead me to a healthy weight? If so, how?

3. What else did I discover from this chapter that I can apply?

How-To Guide
QUICK LIFE HACK
Identify one belief related to weight loss that is holding you back. What is the opposite of that belief? Which of these two beliefs makes more sense? Write down these two beliefs and put them side by side on an index card or somewhere else that is handy. Look at them each day and decide which is true for you.

For a more thorough assessment, complete the exercise below to examine your beliefs and assumptions about losing weight. Then discover a solution that unlocks the door to your success at losing weight and keeping it off.

GUIDEBOOK EXERCISE
Exercise 6: What attitudes and beliefs about weight loss hold you back?

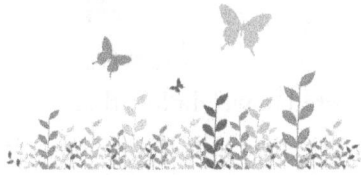

CHAPTER 9

People-Pleasing

PROBLEM: I am afraid to disappoint others.

PRINCIPLE: Connect with what you truly want. Stop wasting time and energy on people pleasing.

How Josie Stopped Being Afraid to Disappoint Others

Remember Josie (from Chapter 6) who had a problem with skipping meals and then overeating at night? One of the things Josie told me was that she loved to get together with her cousin, and they spent three or four hours in a bar enjoying each other's company and drinking beer. She usually drank three or four beers while they were together. Drinking this amount of beer was a roadblock to losing weight. But what would her cousin think of her if she didn't drink beer while they were together? Spending time with her family was a big source of comfort in a difficult time for Josie and she didn't want to cut that time short.

We talked about what to do with her expectation that she should drink beer when she got together with her cousin. She said, "I'm just going to tell him I'm not drinking tonight."

And that's what she did, and they had a great time. When I asked Josie about how she felt about her accomplishment, she told me that she was proud of herself because she had become an advocate for what she really wanted. Josie's choice is a clear example of how to take a stand for yourself. Josie took a positive stand for herself when she stopped people-pleasing so she could connect with what she truly wanted and make her own choices.

My People-Pleasing Story

My memory of being afraid to disappoint others was from when I was a kid. I was anxious about school. I was anxious about getting good grades to make my mom and dad happy with my report cards. My worry, over-responsibility, and people-pleasing continued through my twenty-seven years of public service. Then, I went into business for myself as a dietitian-nutritionist in 2012 to help adults lose weight and keep it off. Seven years ago, I met my business mentor, Heather Dominick, who showed me how to let go of people-pleasing, stop taking things personally, and focus less on what other people think. Instead, I now focus on what really matters to me, what I really want, and what I'm feeling.

Now I'm much more able to determine when I am engaging in people-pleasing and feeling concerned about "what people think." **I am more likely to** say no to clients when it's not a good match instead of wanting their approval. **I am no longer worried** about saying no to the wrong referrals because of what people will think. **I am happy to** go on vacation without taking work with me so I can relax and enjoy my time off. I'm with you on this journey. I'm still building my own ability to say no to people-pleasing.

Problem of Not Wanting to Disappoint Others

This chapter delves into the topic of how to stop people-pleasing and being driven by the need not to disappoint others and what that means for you. Let's dive in. Just what is people-pleasing? People-pleasing as defined here are the actions we take to seek approval. In other words, we behave in ways that we believe will shape what other people think of us. This tendency can start early when, as a child, we begin to figure out what we need to do to fit into our family unit and win approval from our parents. We talk about what people-pleasing can cost us and what we can do instead.

How can you stop being concerned about seeking approval and what other people think? The process of change starts by looking inside at what's in your heart. The key to success at anything worthwhile is heartfelt commitment. As one woman I'm working with said this week with heartfelt conviction, "I've got goals, I know where I'm going."

As Gay Hendricks expressed it in his book, *The Joy of Genius: The Next Step Beyond the Big Leap—a New Way to End Negative Thinking and Liberate Your True Creativity*, "We get what we're committed to getting out of life. We get the positive things we're committing to getting, but you may find, as I did, that you have unconscious commitments that cause you to keep doing things that hurt you." He continues, "Your mind can conceive of a magnificent positive future for you, but your heart is what will make it real."[15]

One of these unconscious commitments can be a concern about what people think of us and a fear of disappointing others that leads to people-pleasing. It's difficult, if not impossible, to be guided by what your heart truly wants when occupied with seeking the approval of others, which can add stress to your life.

How Can You Tell if You're People-Pleasing?

Check in with yourself about these three things if you want to assess whether people-pleasing is part of how you cope:

    a. **Approval seeking:** Do you ask yourself, "What would my wife, parents, boss, friends think about this idea I'm mulling over?"

    b. **You play by someone else's rules:** Do you often hear yourself using the word "should?"
       Example: "I should have a couple of drinks tonight when we get together with friends. If I don't, people will think I'm a party pooper."

    c. **You avoid attention or criticism:** You do things that you don't really want to do because you are afraid of being embarrassed and calling attention to yourself.

If you believe you're not a people-pleaser, take a moment and reflect on how:

✧ Easy or hard it is to say no to requests

✧ You overcame social conditioning

✧ You assess and act on what you really want and what you truly feel

Weight Loss and People-Pleasing

How does people-pleasing apply to your weight loss journey and what can you do about it? A big clue that people-pleasing interferes with your weight loss is to ask yourself whether you are having a difficult time making self-care a priority. If you're taking care of everyone and everything else other than your own self-care and weight loss action goals, it is a sign that your primary focus is on winning approval from others. From my personal and professional experience, people-pleasing can keep your self-care needs as something you'll do after washing and drying the weekly pile of dirty laundry. This preoccupation with people-pleasing can rob you of taking care of yourself, your health, and your well-being.

How Joanne Made Time for Self-Care and Weight Loss

Joanne was a nurse who had worked for the same organization for years. She had a habit of putting her clients and co-workers first. While other staff took their leave and vacations freely, she worked extra hours and on weekends, which left little room for a personal life. Joanne called me at a time when she was getting ready for surgery and needed to lose weight to make the recovery from surgery easier. This upcoming surgery was the reason she was ready to put herself first and take her health seriously. We talked about how she could make room for herself in her life, especially at work.

Joanne decided to begin setting boundaries and saying no to requests that robbed her of time for self-care. She made her own rules about how she would stand up for herself and reclaim her weekends and vacation days. She asked for an assistant, who was hired to help her have a more reasonable workload. One day a week, she found a different office to work in so she could get administrative work done without interruption. She established a lunchtime in the middle of the day when she would eat lunch and then take a walk. Simple changes like this made a huge difference. She lost a significant amount of weight—thirty-eight pounds—before surgery and recovered well. Also, she scheduled a trip to Europe that she'd been wanting to take for years. Saying no to frequent requests for favors helped her to say yes to her new habits of being more physically active and planning what she ate so she could continue to lose weight.

Dr. Robert Kushner, an expert on obesity and creator of Dr. Robert Kushner's Personality Type Diet, developed seven personality types and coping patterns that can become obstacles to weight loss. The people-leaser is one of the coping patterns described in his program guide, which says that having this type of mentality can become an inner obstacle to losing weight. How do you know if you're a people-pleaser? According to Kushner's Coping Lifestyle Patterns Mini-Quiz, a people pleaser is defined as someone who answers yes to this statement: "You keep saying yes to everyone else, which keeps your own needs at the bottom of your 'to do' list."[16]

Why Be Concerned about People-Pleasing?

Dr. Kushner described three important things about people-pleasing that can interfere with weight loss and commitment to self-care:

✧ People-pleasing is a habit that can keep you from self-care.

✧ Self-care is an investment in yourself so you can enjoy your life and be available longer to be there for the people you love.

✧ Your body and mind need to be tuned up and fed the right kind and amount of fuel, just like your car, instead of sputtering and coming to a stop when driven on empty.

People-pleasing is often the biggest thing that keeps us from making ourselves a priority and ultimately our weight loss success, long-term health, and well-being.

Chapter Summary

In this chapter, I delved into the topic of how to stop people-pleasing and being driven by the need to not disappoint others and what that means for you. I gave you a way to assess whether people-pleasing is part of how you cope with stress and whether and how it interferes with your weight loss. I also offered ways to limit people pleasing and let go of what other people think in the Guidebook Exercises.

Companion Chapters for Exploration

Want more help with the problem that you are afraid to disappoint others? Here's a recommended short cut: pick one or more of the chapters below to read next that seem most relevant to you. (These are also listed on the ROADMAP chart in Chapter 4.)

RUNNING ON EMPTY: I DON'T MAKE MYSELF A PRIORITY (CHAPTER 6)

This chapter shows you how to commit daily to declaring your worthiness and making yourself a priority. You are given tips on how to make time for yourself and schedule daily self-care and recognize that self-care is not selfish.

EMPTINESS: I USE FOOD/ALCOHOL AS RELIEF FOR MOOD OR STRESS (CHAPTER 7)

We see that Katie (who we introduced in Chapter 1) reached out for help because when she got angry, sad, and lonely she "stuffed her face" with food. I helped her disrupt this old pattern and consistently apply new habits with my signature process of 5 Steps to Stop Being Controlled by Food.

MINDSET: I DON'T BELIEVE I CAN SUCCEED (CHAPTER 8)

Explore how your mindset and beliefs from the past may interfere with weight loss, and how to cultivate a mindset shift that will help you master new habits.

PERFECTIONISM HOLDS ME BACK: I BEAT MYSELF UP OR GIVE UP IF I DON'T CARRY OUT MY AIMS PERFECTLY (CHAPTER 15)

Judging yourself and beating yourself up are symptoms of perfectionism and cause you to give up on cherished dreams. Curiosity, compassion, and self-acceptance can allow us to make progress instead of being paralyzed by fear of being a failure when we don't carry out our aims flawlessly.

DISCONNECTED: I FORGET ABOUT MY BODY'S NEEDS (CHAPTER 16)

This chapter's purpose is to increase your sense of safety and ability to listen to your body's signals. As you align with your body's feedback, you may notice that it opens the door to trusting that your body's purpose is to protect you.

Reflection Questions

What about you? Here's your opportunity to reflect for a few moments on how people-pleasing applies to you.

1. How does people-pleasing affect my self-care and weight loss intentions? How does it hold me back?

2. When do I have a hard time saying no?

3. What am I willing to do to stop wasting time and energy on what other people think?

How-To Guide

QUICK LIFE HACK

When you use muscles, they grow stronger. Let go of people-pleasing today by saying no at least one time (to something you don't want to do) and strengthen your "no" muscle.

Reportedly, business magnate and investor Warren Buffet said that there is one word that is the most likely to lead to your success. What is that one word? The magic word is: no. The ability to say no to those things that are trivial or less important to you gives you more ability to say yes to the things that are vitally important to you.

GUIDEBOOK EXERCISES

Exercise 7: The Should Exercise
Exercise 8: Letting Go Exercise

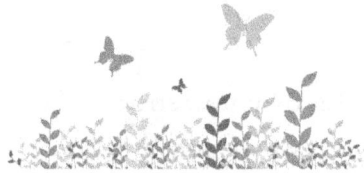

CHAPTER 10

Emptiness

PROBLEM: I use food as a substitute for real fulfillment.

PRINCIPLE: Be guided by what you truly yearn for in life.

Phil's Story

WHEN PHIL FIRST CALLED ME, he told me he didn't believe he could make the changes needed to lose weight and be healthier. He came to me for help because he decided he'd never know what he could do unless he saw in real life whether he could do it. He often found himself taking on extra tasks at work. He sometimes picked up the slack for other people because of his habit of people-pleasing. Afterwards, he felt a sense of emptiness, and wanted a reward. So, he reached for a bag of M&Ms. This habit led him to gain fifty pounds, and then his doctor put him on high blood pressure medication.

Then we partnered together to discover how to disrupt this pattern of eating candy as a reward. When I asked him what was most important to him, he instantly talked about his young daughter. He knew he wanted to be there for her for as long as possible. He didn't like the idea of lying in a hospital bed, dying early, and wishing he had taken better care of himself. Each time he had a craving, he stopped and asked himself, "Is it worth it? Is it worth it to not eat this candy right now so I'll be able to see my daughter grow up?"

That's how Phil tapped into what was important to him and how he made a change in what he ate that supported what he valued the most.

Do you know what's missing for you and what it is that you truly want? It may be a lost dream that is lying dormant, or a wish to nurture an important relationship like it was for Phil. Or maybe you want to fulfill a desire for adventure that's on your life bucket list. Ignoring what you truly long for can lead you to overeat as a cheap substitute for living the life you've always wanted to live. This is a life where you are healthy in mind and body at the weight you want to be and you look in the mirror and love who you see and do the things you've always wanted to do.

How to Infuse Your Life with Joy, Purpose, and Meaning

If you aren't in touch with what gives your life purpose and meaning, you may be missing out on what can make you flourish and instead using food as a consolation. It may be time to rediscover what's important. It can be easier than you think to find simple ways, like Phil did, to take your life from feelings of boredom to joy. As you seek joy, meaning, and purpose, think beyond food—especially if food has become a substitute for what matters in life. Let's take a journey of discovery together and explore what you truly want that will help motivate you to change habits and lose weight—and keep it off.

Advertising Gimmicks

Beware of advertisements that promise happiness from buying, eating, or drinking any food product. Examples of such ads are ones that suggest that you can "open happiness" as you twist off the top of a bottle of soda or eat a bag of potato chips with the tagline, "Happiness is Simple." Recently I saw a box for a slice of pizza that read, "Slice of Happiness."

One thing we know for sure is that happiness and thriving don't come in a bottle or in a package of processed food. Why grasp at straws and go for instant gratification that lets us down for a few brief minutes? Although eating is highly pleasurable, we all know in our heart of hearts that what we eat is not all of or even at the center of what gives our life meaning. Maybe it's time to let go of feeling like you live to eat.

How to Discover What Gives Your Life Purpose and Meaning

You're here reading this book for a reason, and you want to have a different outcome this time. You can shed excess weight and keep it off. But how, you ask? It takes more than cutting calories and increasing physical activity temporarily to achieve lasting weight loss success. It takes a mindset transformation, as discussed in Chapter 8, and knowing what you truly yearn for to produce the motivation, focus, and resilience to get your results. Even though motivation, focus, and resilience can't be bought, you can find them by looking within. You can experience a joyful journey in the process.

This chapter will examine the topic of what it will take for you to flourish and how being at a healthy weight will contribute to that. Martin Seligman, founder of positive psychology, professor of psychology at the University of Pennsylvania, and author, wrote in his book, *Flourish*, that to flourish is about much more than positive emotions that drive life satisfaction. It takes a life filled with well-being to flourish according to Seligman. Let's look at Seligman's five Elements of Well-Being:[17]

   ✧   Positive emotion

   ✧   Engagement

   ✧   Meaning

   ✧   Accomplishment

   ✧   Positive relationships

The first element of well-being, defined as positive emotion in Seligman's book, is the foundation for being in a good mood, life satisfaction, and happiness. Engagement, the second element, is represented by activities that absorb us with rapt attention. The third element of meaning he defined as dedication to something bigger than yourself. Accomplishments translate to achievement and mastery. Finally, the elements of positive relationships are central as a motivating force for almost everyone.

What Gives Your Life Purpose and Meaning?

In this chapter, you are asked to reflect on what gives your life purpose and meaning, especially if you use food as a substitute for true fulfillment. The most relevant question is: what is your desired contribution to others and serving something bigger than yourself?

If you aren't sure what gives your life meaning, it may be time to rediscover what matters most.

Chapter Summary

What matters to you most? That is the thing that gets you out of bed in the morning besides a job, family, and the needs of pets. This chapter is designed to help you hone in on what it is you really yearn for. In a busy life, it's easy to forget what's truly important, give into cravings, and grab a salty, fatty, or sweet processed snack instead of reaching for what you truly want in life.

Companion Chapters for Exploration

Want more help with the problem that you use food as a substitute for real fulfillment? Here's a recommended short cut: pick one or more of the chapters below to read next that seem most relevant to you. (These are also listed on the ROADMAP chart in Chapter 4.)

RUNNING ON EMPTY: I DON'T MAKE MYSELF A PRIORITY (CHAPTER 6)

This chapter demonstrates how to commit daily to declaring your worthiness and making yourself a priority. I share with you how to make time for yourself and schedule daily self-care and to recognize that self-care is not selfish.

SELF-SOOTHING: I USE FOOD/ALCOHOL AS RELIEF FOR MOOD OR STRESS (CHAPTER 7)

We see that Katie (who we introduced in Chapter 1) reached out for help because when she got angry, sad, and lonely she "stuffed her face" with food. I helped her disrupt this old pattern and consistently apply new habits with our signature process of Five Steps to Stop Being Controlled by Food.

MOTIVATION: I LOSE TRACK OF WHY WEIGHT LOSS MATTERS (CHAPTER 11)

In this chapter, I emphasize how easy it is to lose sight of your why—that is, why weight loss matters. Instead, you are given helpful ways to get and stay motivated during your weight loss journey. You are also shown how to keep your reasons to lose weight in full sight. You are asked to envision the kind of person you want to become and change conflicting beliefs that can help you stay focused during your weight loss journey.

FEELING STUCK: I DON'T KNOW WHY I KEEP REPEATING OLD PATTERNS (CHAPTER 13)

It's far easier to repeat old patterns when we aren't present in the moment and are unconscious of the choices we are making. In this chapter I share how to heal the past, embrace the present, and choose your future.

**INSPIRING ACTION: I START OUT STRONG,
THEN I LOSE MOMENTUM (CHAPTER 17)**

This chapter builds on the question of, "How can you keep up your momentum once you discover your top motivators for a happy life at a healthy weight?" In this chapter I share that a big secret to weight loss success is inspired daily commitment, which we call recommitment.

Reflection Questions

Answer these reflection questions to help you focus on what it is you really yearn for instead of using food as a consolation prize:

1. Give an example of what in your life makes you flourish and experience well-being?

2. What does it look and feel like to live this kind of life?

3. How will being at a healthy weight contribute?

How-To Guide

LIFE HACK

What are five things you've always wanted to do? With whom do you want to share these things and why?

GUIDEBOOK EXERCISES

Exercise 9: On Purpose and Meaning

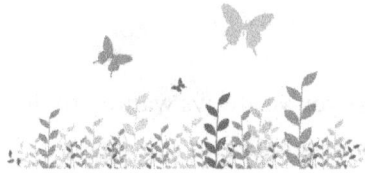

CHAPTER 11

Motivation

PROBLEM: I lose sight of why weight loss matters.

PRINCIPLE: Discover your prime motivator for weight loss.

SOME PEOPLE ARE ESPECIALLY GOOD at starting new projects like weight loss. Then, after a few weeks, their progress slows because they lose sight of why weight loss matters and they give up on themselves. Why is this? Sometimes initial motivation wanes in the process of doing what it takes to put new habits into practice consistently. We lose sight of the fact that good things take time.

When Michelle first called me, she told me that she was frustrated with her nutrition and weight-related health problems like back and knee pain and elevated blood sugar that indicated that she was pre-diabetic. All this was compounded by stressful life situations. Her husband had been sick for years and had passed away and her son was having a hard time. She also had suffered a childhood trauma.

Michelle wanted help because she was using food to manage her mood and stress and her health was suffering from it. She aimed to lose sixty pounds to get back her health and mobility. She wanted to do the outdoors activities she loved like hiking, kayaking, and cycling. She yearned to feel more confident in her body and how she interacted with the world by losing weight. It was time to start her life again: she had just moved to a place she liked in the greater Washington, D.C. area. One belief that complicated her commitment to losing weight was that she associated losing weight with illness because her husband's illness had caused him to lose weight.

We did an assessment and created a plan and Michelle started out well. She lost sixteen pounds in four months by walking consistently, eating more fruits and vegetables, and eating out less often, especially at fast food restaurants. She worked at home during the pandemic and that helped her make healthy lifestyle changes. Then a series of things happened to her, including returning to the workplace after the pandemic, which caused her to lose sight of her body's needs and why weight loss mattered. To celebrate going back to work, her company hosted lots of after-work parties to welcome employees back to the workspace. Michelle felt the need to fit in at work, and soon she lost sight of her motivation to lose weight.

To compound matters, she contracted an illness that sapped her strength. Once well again, she visited her family, and that had stirred up memories from past trauma. Then she got COVID-19 and it took months for her to recover. For all these reasons, she was distracted and had a difficult time focusing on weight loss and what mattered most. All the while she began to regain weight.

Recently, Michelle reached out to resume her weight loss sessions with me. She has started walking two miles a day and has begun losing weight again with a new awareness of how easy it is to forget her intentions to change the behaviors it takes to lose weight. She also is aware of her tendency to forget about her body's needs while at work and a pattern of skipping meals during the day. She is countering this tendency to skip meals by packing a lunch the night before and bringing it with her and has put a thirty-minute lunch break on her calendar to help her remember to eat lunch. Michelle also is eating breakfast before she goes to work. Now she is in the process of losing weight again and is armed with renewed motivation and awareness of why weight loss matters and what can get in the way.

Why Weight Loss Matters

Because it's easy to lose sight of why weight loss matters, it makes a difference when we keep our reasons for wanting to lose weight front and center. How do we keep our eyes on why we want to lose weight during our weight loss journey? This chapter takes a look at helpful ways to tap into your weight loss and keep your reasons to lose weight in full sight.

Motivation

How can you "get motivated" to embark on your weight loss journey and have the grit to stay with it? Perhaps what's missing is awareness of your weight loss "why." Research on motivation shows that for projects requiring significant creativity, a "carrot and stick" system of rewards and punishments may backfire. Extrinsic or external rewards may dampen motivation, according to research cited by Daniel Pink in his book *Drive: The Surprising Truth About What Motivates Us*.[18]

Intrinsic or internal motivators have more staying power than extrinsic motivators in the long run according to Pink. Intrinsic motivators promote greater physical and mental well-being based on research cited by Pink in his insightful book. Intrinsic motivation is self-directed, requires engagement, and aligns with what gives your life meaning. People often come to me for help who are seeking a way to discover the motivation needed to lose weight and keep it off. The golden key is to connect weight loss to what matters most in your life.

This chapter is designed for you to tap into your innate motivation to lose weight as we explore how to build a shame-free, healthy relationship with food. Michelle shared her intrinsic motivation to lose weight when she told me how her health was suffering because of her weight gain. This prompted her desire to improve her health and mobility so she can do the outdoor activities that she always loved.

Fuel Your Motivation by Making Changes from the Inside Out

In his book *Atomic Habits,* James Clear revealed a new way to look at why the challenge of changing habits is difficult and how to avoid the biggest mistakes we make as we try to change habits that cause us to lose our way. He explained that we focus on the wrong things and try to implement change in the wrong way. He identified three layers of behavior change and noted that we usually begin in the wrong place. These three layers focus on where to start with the habit change process. Clear recommended starting on the inside instead of focusing on the outside with the outcome because ultimately it is less effective.

3 Layers of Behavior Change

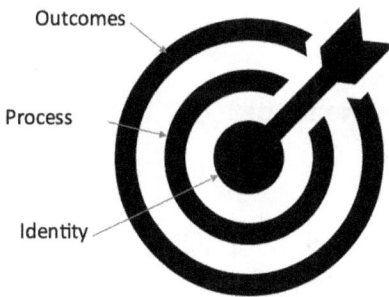

Outcomes

Process

Identity

Atomic Habits, An Easy & Proven Way to Build Good Habits & Break Bad Ones by James Clear

Identifying the Kind of Person You Want to Be

According to Clear, we make a mistake when we focus first on outcomes we want to achieve when taking action to change habits. Clear suggested instead that we can be more successful and sustain new habits and when we begin with the inside layer that represents our identity. Clarifying your beliefs about what you want in life can be a good place to start and is an important part of clarifying who you want to become. It's easy to set up desires that are in conflict with each other. For example, Robert, a self-employed entrepreneur, wanted to lose weight, but he didn't take action on this desired outcome because he believed he'd have to go hungry to succeed and said, "I don't want to starve myself."

Let's take a new look at where to start the change process in a simple way that you can easily remember. Let's start on the inside and imagine your future, then make changes from the inside out. When looking inside, you have the ability to reflect on your mindset, beliefs, and desires. Figure 2 shows a different way of looking at the steps involved in behavior change with a three step BE–DO–HAVE. behavior change approach.

STEP 1: BE. → STEP 2: DO. → STEP 3: HAVE.

What does each step mean, practically speaking?

STEP 1: BE.
Who do you want to BE (you feeling fulfilled with supportive beliefs)?

STEP 2: DO.
What will you DO to make this happen?

STEP 3: HAVE.
What results do you want to HAVE?

Jeanette's Vision for the Future

Remember when we talked about Jeanette in Chapter 8 on Mindset? Jeanette's story is a beautiful example of how powerful it can be to start with changing your beliefs and what kind of a person you want to BE. Then, the next steps are to create a plan for what you'll DO to make this happen and achieve the results you want to HAVE. When Jeanette first called me, she said, "I want to become an example of healthy aging."

What she meant by that declaration was that she wanted to become active and healthy as she aged. Envisioning herself as an example of healthy aging was timely for Jeanette because she was just about to turn sixty years old. Using her vision to guide her actions helped her to apply patience, determination, and motivation to eat healthier and become physically active.

Chapter Summary

This chapter emphasized how easy it is to lose sight of why weight loss matters, and this problem makes it even more important to keep our reasons in focus for wanting to lose weight. Included in this chapter are helpful ways to get and stay motivated during your weight loss journey. You are shown how beneficial it is to keep your reasons to lose weight in full sight. You are then asked to envision the kind of person you want to become and change conflicting beliefs so you can stay focused on building momentum during your weight loss journey.

Companion Chapters for Exploration

Want more help with the problem that you lose track of why weight loss matters? Here's a recommended shortcut: pick one or more of the chapters below to read next that seem most relevant to you. (These are also listed on the ROADMAP chart in Chapter 4.)

MOTIVATION: I DON'T BELIEVE I CAN SUCCEED (CHAPTER 8)

Together we explore how your mindset and beliefs from the past may interfere with weight loss, and how to cultivate a mindset shift that will help you master new habits.

EMPTINESS: I USE FOOD AS A SUBSTITUTE FOR REAL FULFILLMENT (CHAPTER 10)

This chapter examines how ignoring what you truly long for can lead to overeating as a cheap substitute for living the life you've always wanted to live and how you can be guided by what you truly yearn for. In the How-To Guide section we point you to an exercise designed to help you to discover what gives your life purpose and meaning.

RUNNING ON EMPTY: DAILY STRESS OR LACK OF SLEEP LEAVE ME TOO TIRED FOR SELF-CARE (CHAPTER 14)

In this chapter we introduce you to the whys and ways to leave behind fatigue caused by stress and lack of sleep so you can live the life you want to live—a happy life at a healthy weight.

INSPIRING ACTION: I START OUT STRONG, THEN I LOSE MOMEN-TUM (CHAPTER 17)

This chapter builds on the question of: How can you keep up your momentum once you've discovered your top motivators for a happy life at a healthy weight? In this chapter we share that a big secret to weight loss success is inspired daily commitment that we call recommitment.

BUILDING CONFIDENCE: I'M AFRAID OF FAILING OR SUCCEEDING AT WEIGHT LOSS (CHAPTER 18)

Are you afraid when you think about losing weight? In this chapter we focus on how fear can easily lead to self-sabotage and sidetrack you from your intentions. Instead, I recommend that you focus on the things you can change as you make lifestyle choices that will support you on your weight loss journey. Then we offer ways to choose your future with a change process and ways you can choose your response to events for a better outcome.

Reflection Questions

Let's conclude our exploration of how to fuel weight loss motivation with these reflection questions:

1. What does your desired vision of the future look like and who do you want to be?

2. What is an important and motivating reason for you to lose weight and keep it off?

3. How will losing weight and making lifestyle changes support you in becoming the kind of person you want to be?

Take a few moments to reflect on each of these three questions to help you get in touch with your innate motivation that can act as a springboard to your successful weight loss journey. Then, complete the exercise in the How-To Guide.

How-To Guide

QUICK LIFE HACK

Ask yourself how losing weight will contribute to your physical, emotional, and mental well-being.

GUIDEBOOK EXERCISE

Exercise 10: Fueling Your Weight Loss Motivation

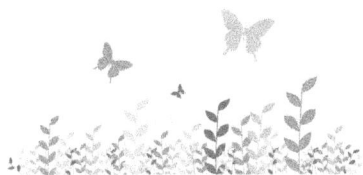

CHAPTER 12

Lack of Consistency

PROBLEM: Lack of Consistency: new habits fall by the wayside.

PRINCIPLE: Build new habits. Act daily with consistency.

Michelle's New Habit

Remember Michelle from Chapter 11 and her series of life events that drained her motivation and made her forget why weight loss mattered? One event that caused her to slip up was a holiday visit to her family. After she came back, she fell into an old habit of eating dinner in front of the TV while she ate comfort food and binge-watched old favorite programs. This visit had brought up old family memories that upset her and reminded her of the causes of childhood shame. The result? She stuffed down her unwanted feelings by making and eating comfort foods that her grandmother used to make for her. She ate from the time she turned on the TV until she went to bed.

Living out this Food-Shame Cycle every night, she began regaining the hard-won weight she had just lost. Her knees began to ache again.

Then, when we worked through the Five Step Process to Stop Being Controlled by Food, she discovered her solution. As a result, Michelle realized that when she turned on the TV, it triggered her to go into automatic pilot and eat her way through the evening. Instead, she changed this unhealthy habit. She decided instead to make a healthier meal and sit down and eat at the dinner table at 6:30 p.m. The side benefit was that her son sat down with her and they had good conversations. Michelle made this new habit consistent and easy to remember by linking dinner to a specific location and time. The key to her making this change was that she no longer automatically turned on the TV before dinner.

Change Habits and Build a Healthy Relationship with Food

In this chapter, you'll learn how to build new and sustainable habits with consistency. These new habits will help you successfully lose weight and keep it off. If you focus your attention with the right mindset and actions, your hard work will bear fruit. In this chapter I build on this latest brain research and habit change techniques to help you build consistency—the defining ingredient to your success at creating a happy life at a healthy weight. The problem is that the rational brain (the neocortex) is the newest part of the brain. It easily goes offline when we are stressed. Then the emotional brain can interfere with our food choices, and it's easier to revert to prior unhealthy habits. We are up against a big challenge when we decide to build new, healthier habits.

It may seem obvious that it takes a focused mind to lose weight and keep it off. But just what is a focused mind? It means using sustained attention and an intentional process to move in the direction of your goals with aware, conscious choices.

A flexible structure, process, and plan that is sustainable makes for long-term success. This comprehensive lifestyle change program is designed to empower you to make better choices by changing your habits. It's not a diet with strict requirements. Instead, you are offered a flexible structure that allows you to eat anything you want selectively by paying attention to how much and how often you eat specific foods, especially when they are processed foods that are high in calories, salt, saturated fat, and sugar.

Creating A New Habit: Where Consistency Starts

Begin building consistency one new habit at a time. How do you create a new habit? Awareness is the starting gate of habit change. The first step is to define what new habits you'll need to become who you want to be—the kind of person who has a healthy relationship with food. The next step is to develop a process to get there. Let's start by looking at one habit you want to change. Choose a pesky habit that is getting in the way of your progress and ask yourself this question:

What is one specific habit you want to change that will help you lose weight? Be specific. For example: eat a smaller amount of food at dinner.

How an Existing Unhelpful Habit Operates

Do you know how the habit you just decided to change operates in your life? Let's look at what usually happens when you make an unhelpful choice. Noticing the actual habit as you play it out in real time when it surfaces makes it more real according to James Clear, author of *Atomic Habits*, who suggested explaining the bad habit out loud as you do it.[19]

Consider a Cookie Habit Example

For example, you might say out loud, "I am now sitting in front of the TV digging into a box of cookies and I might actually eat the whole box. If I do, I'm going to feel good for a few minutes and then I'm going to beat myself up for making this unconscious choice."

By intentionally noticing behavior that is usually unconscious, you have begun the process of letting go of having food control you. Once you have completed this exercise for yourself, you can become aware of a specific food you crave, like a box of cookies, and how it usually plays out. You can couple this new awareness with the Five Step Process to Stop Letting Food Control You instead of going on auto-pilot and eating mindlessly. (See Chapter 7.)

Starting a New Habit

What else can you do once you've defined the habit you want to change and are aware of the consequences? The best way to start a new habit is to make your new, healthier habit easy to remember and use by linking it to a specific time and location just like Michelle did to curb overeating after dinner as mentioned earlier in the chapter. Another easy hack is to link a new habit that you intend to adopt to another well-established habit. Take Max, one of my clients, who chewed gum after meals to keep from overeating.

Discover the Environmental and Social Cues to Overeating

Let's look at habit change in a different way using behavior change theory. Are you tired of eating handfuls of candy or other foods when you're not even hungry and simply eating mindlessly? Learned environmental and social cues can encourage unconscious eating. How can you change these cues and behaviors? Three of the most effective ways for creating behavior change are:

1. Change the environment
2. Eliminate the cue
3. Separate the cue from eating

Change the environment: Ever notice that when food is visible and within reach that you are more likely to eat it without thinking?

You can change the environment by making foods and beverages that you plan to eat more of within easy reach and put foods that you plan to eat less of out of sight (or out of the house). In our house we always have a bowl of fruit on the counter, which makes this healthy snack visible and within reach.

Eliminate the cue: You can avoid tempting foods at the office or at a religious service by pouring your cup of coffee and then immediately moving away from the area where food is served.

Separate the cue from eating: It helps to break the mindless eating cycle when you make eating off limits in certain situations, for example, while watching television.

Notice that Michelle, in her example above, decided to disassociate the cue of turning on the TV before dinner to break the chain of unhelpful behaviors and overeating in the evening.

HOW TO STICK WITH GOOD HABITS

The hardest part of being successful with weight loss or any project is that it requires continued effort and attention. In contrast, bad habits are easy to slide into like eating chips or ice cream in front of the TV at night after a stressful day. It can be a challenge to keep up new, healthy habits because the older unhealthy habits are so well ingrained. What can you do to keep new habits going?

How Can You Make Tracking Fun?

The number one practice for weight loss success is tracking progress by monitoring what you eat and drink. There is solid evidence that it works when you track and monitor what you consume. I recommend that you use an app for tracking what you eat to make it quick and easy. With the MyNetDiary app, I recommend, you can complete daily food tracking in as little as five minutes a day. The act of monitoring your food and beverage intake makes you aware of what you eat and drink and can give you a sense of satisfaction.

How can you turn tracking into a game? When you mark your achievements on your ROADMAP Action Plan, it can bring you the reward and satisfaction that you've accomplished something important. You can make it fun when you notice that you are on a winning streak as you check off accomplishments. Even if you stumble and forget to record your food and drink, you can feel a sense of satisfaction when you get back on track.

Now we've introduced why tracking your food and drink can help you stay on a winning streak, let's consider ways to build consistency with evidence of your accomplishments. Create a visual reminder of your day's accomplishments at the end of the day, by putting a checkmark next to each action goal completed. As one of my clients, Daphne, told me, "I'm in competition with myself, and that's why I record my accomplishments each day. It helps me feel good about the walk I took and my food choices."

When you track your progress with habit change, it can be exciting enough to want to keep that winning streak going as James Clear noted in *Atomic Habits*.[20] He also shared devices to make progress visible and satisfying including what he called "The Paper Clip Strategy." Clear reported the story of an inexperienced stockbroker who measured his progress each time he made a sales call. After each call, he moved a paper clip from one jar that was initially filled with 120 paper clips to an empty jar. He continued making calls until all paper clips had been moved from one jar to the other and with this new habit, he became enormously successful. Why not create your own fun and simple way to make your progress satisfying?

Hint for Success with Eating and Consistency

Here are words to live by so you can eat any foods you want selectively and still lose weight.

Do I Have to Put Certain Foods Off-Limits?

Changing your response to certain cues doesn't mean that you can't eat your favorite foods. Instead, plan for what, when, and how much you'll eat these foods selectively and then savor them without guilt.

Chapter Summary

In this chapter we've covered how to define a habit you want to change and become aware of the consequences of this habit. We've also shown you how to address the environmental and social cues of overeating and make new habits stick by turning tracking new habits into a game.

Companion Chapters for Exploration

Want more help with the problem that you apply new habits, then they fall by the wayside? Here's a recommended shortcut: pick one or more of the chapters below to read next that seem most relevant to you. (These are also listed on the ROADMAP chart in Chapter 4.)

SELF-SOOTHING: I USE FOOD/ALCOHOL AS RELIEF FOR MOOD OR STRESS (CHAPTER 7)

We see that Katie, who was introduced in Chapter 1, reached out for help because when she got angry, sad, and lonely she "stuffed her face" with food. She was able to disrupt this old pattern and consistently apply new habits with my signature process of Five Steps to Stop Being Controlled by Food.

MINDSET: I DON'T BELIEVE I CAN SUCCEED (CHAPTER 8)

Together we explore how your mindset and beliefs from the past may interfere with weight loss, and how to cultivate a mindset shift that will help you build consistency and master new habits.

MOTIVATION: I LOSE TRACK OF WHY WEIGHT LOSS MATTERS (CHAPTER 11)

This chapter emphasizes how easy it is to lose sight of your why—that is, why weight loss matters. Instead, you are given helpful ways to get and stay motivated during your weight loss journey. I also show you how to keep your reasons to lose weight in full sight to help you act consistency to change habits. You are asked to envision the kind of person you want to be and change conflicting beliefs that can help you stay focused during your weight loss journey.

INSPIRING ACTION: I START OUT STRONG, THEN I LOSE MOMEN-TUM (CHAPTER 17)

How can you keep up your momentum and consistency once you've discovered your top motivators for a happy life at a healthy weight? In this chapter we share that a big secret to weight loss success is inspired daily commitment that we call recommitment.

BUILDING CONFIDENCE: I'M AFRAID OF FAILING OR SUCCEEDING AT WEIGHT LOSS (CHAPTER 18)

Are you afraid when you think about losing weight? In this chapter, we focus on how fear can easily lead to self-sabotage and sidetrack you from your intentions. Instead, I recommend that you focus on the things you can change as you make lifestyle choices that will support you on your weight loss journey. Then you are offered ways to choose your future with a change process and ways you can choose your response to events for a better outcome.

Reflection Questions

1. Once you've decided on a habit to change, ask yourself, "How can I turn this intention into consistent action in support of my weight loss journey?"

2. How can I make this new habit stick by making it easy to remember and do?

How-To Guide

LIFE HACK

If you're physically hungry, choose a low-calorie food that is bulky and filling like a bowl of vegetable soup, a piece of fruit, a 100-calorie bag of popcorn, or a cup of tea as another way to break the habit of eating high calorie snacks in front of the TV.

Monitor what you do. Mindfully track your food, drink, physical activities and other action goals to become more aware of and give yourself credit for what you're doing. This awareness can help you identify which actions are helpful and what you're doing or not doing that is holding you back.

GUIDEBOOK EXERCISES

Resource 1: ROADMAP Daily Action Plan: Tracking Your Progress

Exercise 11: Changing Your Response to Environmental and Social Cues

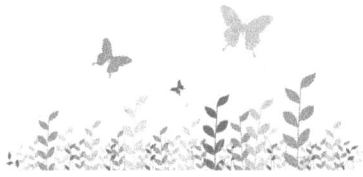

CHAPTER 13

Feeling Stuck

PROBLEM: I don't know why I keep repeating old patterns.

PRINCIPLE: Let go of old habits and survival mechanisms. Heal the past, embrace the present, and choose your future.

Max's Story of Repeating Old Patterns

I was sitting in my office one day when Max, a high-level mid-career professional, called me. He told me that he had gained weight after he was excluded from a military post because he was too heavy to meet the weight requirement. He was so disappointed with this rejection that he ate fast food at every meal and gained 200 pounds in two years. He had many health problems because of this weight gain and said that he got out of breath when he walked from the parking lot to his desk at work. He knew that if he didn't do something to change his lifestyle, he would have even more serious health issues. Max was continuing an old pattern of using food to handle disappointments and rejection.

We did an assessment and created a lifestyle change plan focused on healthy eating, smaller amounts of food at meals, and increased physical activity to lose weight. He tracked what he ate using the smartphone app I recommended. He began swimming almost daily for more than an hour and realized that his weight loss journey wasn't a sprint but a marathon. During the year Max worked with me, he lost weight consistently, and at the end of the year he had lost 120 pounds and was committed to continuing to lose weight. He had decided for himself that he wanted and needed to lose weight and intended to be alert to future disappointments and handle them in such a way that he could stay committed to his health and be true to himself.

If you find yourself feeling stuck by repeating old patterns and habits from the past, it may be time to heal the past, embrace the present, and choose your future just like Max did.

Embracing the Present Moment

Being conscious in the present moment is the key to freeing yourself from being bogged down by the past or being worried about a potential unwanted situation in the future. When you're absorbed in the present moment, fear can't take hold. Freedom is what comes from realizing that the present moment is all there is. Being in the present can help you to be light-hearted and to seize the moment you're in with your sense of humor intact instead of being wrapped up in worry and anxiety about the past or future.

Planning and preparing for your vision of the future is part of your ROADMAP to Success and an activity that can fully absorb you. Being in the present moment doesn't mean you can't prepare for the future and that you are just "taking things as they come." Planning ahead to anticipate roadblocks is key to success on this kind of journey. Without planning and/or packing your lunch ahead of time, for example, it can be an easy default response to eat something quickly from the cafeteria, get takeout, or stop by a fast food or casual dining restaurant and overeat.

Being in the present with a sense of being "in flow" (absorbed in the moment) is a natural extension of choosing love instead of fear. Love is expansive. On the other hand, fear can make you contract and then pull away, withdraw, or hide. Fear can result from thinking about potential negative consequences associated with the past or future.

How do we enjoy the present moment when there are so many pressures to contend with in life? Many tools for living more fully in the present come from simple practices that help us switch from a stress to a relaxation response. These tools help us slow down and take care of ourselves in a busy world. Practices like meditation, breathing, yoga, T'ai Chi, and physical activity can bring us back to a state of relaxation and equanimity and connect us with the present moment. Slowing down while eating is another good way to be present in the moment. This week I'm finding that I become totally absorbed in the moment when I read passages from inspirational books like *The Book of Joy, Lasting Happiness in a Changing World* by His Holiness the Dalai Lama, Archbishop Desmond Tutu, and Douglas Abrams.

What Gets in the Way

What gets in the way of living in the present and at what cost? Over-eating is just one behavior that can lead us away from living the life we want to live. Buddhism is concerned with the suffering that is caused when we are caught up in desire and cravings or avoidance based on a past event and fear of the future. A quote, often attributed to the Dalai Lama, describes this problem well. In response to being asked what surprises him most, the Dalai Lama replied, "Man, because he sacrifices his health to make money. Then he sacrifices money to recuperate his health. And then he is so anxious about the future that he does not enjoy the present; the result being that he does not live in the present or the future. He lives as if he is never going to die, and then dies having never really lived."

I love this explanation of how we tie ourselves in knots in life as we give up our present enjoyment and health, which is what makes us whole, to pursue money, career, and status. Then, we turn around and invest in repairing the health that we've lost. The problem is that we don't enjoy the present as we put our health at risk for our career or to make money and this is how we end up in burnout and exhaustion. When we can enjoy the present and take care of the health we have, while being productive and creative, this is the very definition of work-life balance. Living the life you want to live is the reason that we encourage you to stop repeating the past and start enjoying the present moment. It isn't inevitable to sacrifice your health and well-being and curtail your years of an active, healthy life.

How and why would you want to live more of your time in the present? A big problem related to our health and weight is that most of us don't make lifestyle choices intentionally and instead make unconscious choices that put our well-being and health at risk. When you are aware of the present moment it is easier to disrupt old patterns so you can take a stand, empower yourself, and actively choose how you want to live and make supportive lifestyle choices.

Healing the Past

Events from the past can leave a residue that can cause us to worry and have feelings of shame and regret that persist and affect our whole life, including our food choices. Some challenges are easier to overcome than others, especially when there's a hidden commitment involved.

Immunity to Change

Why is change so hard and what can we do about it? According to Robert Kegan and Lisa Laskow Lahey, authors of *Immunity to Change: How to Overcome it and Unlock the Potential in Yourself and Your Organization,* straightforward challenges are easily handled when they are technical problems[21] These are problems that can be handled with a simple "how to" plan that is a quick and easy solution to challenges. It's easy for some people to lose weight, especially people who only need to lose those extra ten pounds. They simply use a formula like a diet that works well for them in the long run. Most of the time though, weight problems aren't a technical problem and simple methods like dieting don't work. Authors Kegan and Lahey point out that with most adults, many challenges, including weight loss, are more complex adaptive changes and require that we adapt and transform our mindset, a topic explored in Chapter 8.

Do you believe that the reason why we resist change is that it makes us feel uncomfortable? In *Immunity to Change*, Kegan and Lahey refute this popular belief. One of their major premises is that the difficulty with change is that most of these challenges are adaptive issues rather than technical problems. The authors wrote that with adaptive challenges, we protect ourselves against the possibility that we will "feel defenseless in the face of dangers and that is what causes us anxiety."[22] The answer? We can overturn "a bad bargain" that we made with ourselves according to the authors because our system of protective behaviors or immunity to change "has been giving us relief from anxiety while creating a false belief that many things are impossible for us to do—things that are completely possible for us to do."

How does this bad bargain work? Kegan and Lahey suggested that we often have hidden commitments that compete with what we say we want. The authors cited three examples of hidden commitments that confound our weight loss success. These hidden commitments can upend our weight loss aspirations and cause us to overeat instead of acting on our intention to eat less and for a compelling reason. These reasons include these wishes:

1. For stimulation and from boredom.
2. To no longer feel empty inside.
3. Not to be seen or treated like a sex object.

I remember being caught in this kind of cross-current. For years I hid by being overweight to avoid unwanted attention. One time when I had lost weight as an adult, I recall being upset when I heard unnerving cat calls from men as I walked down the street. I didn't want to be seen as a sex object. This incident reminded me that I had a hidden commitment to avoid attention from men and being seen as a sex object. It took courage to face this fear and take a stand for myself to transform these old patterns and hidden commitments and create a shame-free healthy relationship with food.

Default Rules

What else can you do to heal the past so you can choose your future intentionally? Meghan Lucas offers insights into how to take a stand for yourself, let go of the past, and make your own rules in her book *Dear Strong Woman, You Make the Rules: How to Rewrite the Rules You Live By, So You Can Live Life on Your Terms.*[23] Lucas brilliantly shows women how to identify the default rules that can hold them back from living the life they want to live. She revealed how to create a new path and a vision to rewrite your own rules for the future.

Default rules come in all shapes and sizes. It wasn't surprising to see a response from one of Lucas's clients to a question about default rules. Her client said that her default rule was, "A thin body is a healthy body. The smaller you are, the more idolized you will be."

Lucas also asked in her book about how we can rewrite our default rules so they are freeing and lead us to who we truly are instead of replacing one set of restrictions with another. Lucas further noted that rewriting your default rules brings uncertainty and a willingness to allow yourself to explore new terrain. Ah, the idea of allowing that discomfort can mean progress at returning home to who you truly are.

I love that Lucas starts with the idea to trust your intuition to get started on the path to convert default rules into empowering behaviors. These are behaviors that move you to the life you want to live. What a beautiful idea of letting go of the old and then letting in the new that brings you home to your magnificent self.

What old patterns and default rules may be preventing your weight loss success? Let's look further and explore how to become aware of what is driving you to repeat old patterns and what you can do to disrupt them.

Chapter Summary

The purpose of this chapter is to team up with you to help you let go of fears that hold you back so you can free yourself from old patterns that are so easy to keep repeating, especially when it comes to overeating. We start with the importance of embracing the present moment to make conscious lifestyle choices and eat consciously to find fulfillment without overeating so you can build a healthy relationship with food. Letting go of the past and being in the present moment lays the foundation for choosing your future—the life you want to live—a happy life at a healthy weight.

Companion Chapters for Exploration

Want more help with the problem that you don't know why you keep repeating old patterns? Here's a recommended shortcut: pick one or more of the chapters below to read next that seem most relevant to you. (These are also listed on the ROADMAP chart in Chapter 4.)

SELF-SOOTHING: I USE FOOD/ALCOHOL AS RELIEF FOR MOOD OR STRESS (CHAPTER 7)

We see that Katie, who was introduced in Chapter 1, reached out for help because when she got angry, sad, and lonely she "stuffed her face" with food. She was able to disrupt this old pattern and consistently apply new habits with my signature process of Five Steps to Stop Being Controlled by Food.

MINDSET: I DON'T BELIEVE I CAN SUCCEED (CHAPTER 8)

This chapter Explores how your mindset and beliefs from the past may interfere with weight loss, and how to cultivate a mindset shift that will help you master new habits.

PEOPLE-PLEASING: I'M AFRAID TO DISAPPOINT OTHERS (CHAPTER 9)

People-pleasing causes us to trim our sails in life about what's possible because we are worried about what other people think and with winning their acceptance and approval instead of scheduling time for self-care. This chapter addresses what you can do about people-pleasing and what other people think.

BUILDING CONFIDENCE: I'M AFRAID OF FAILING OR SUCCEEDING AT WEIGHT LOSS (CHAPTER 18)

Are you afraid when you think about losing weight? In this chapter, we focus on how fear can easily lead to self-sabotage and sidetrack you from your intentions. Instead, the chapter focuses on the things you can change as you make better lifestyle choices. Then, you can choose your future with a change process and ways you can choose your response to events for a better outcome.

TUNED OUT: MY LIFESTYLE CHOICES ARE LARGELY UNCONSCIOUS (CHAPTER 19)

For many of us, lifestyle choices are largely unconscious and that causes us to overeat and forget about self-care. We are given essential advantages and aspects of making conscious choices, including paying attention while we eat and slowing down enough so we can tell when we're full without overeating.

Letting go of fear and freeing yourself from the past sets the foundation for taking a stand for yourself and empowering yourself to accept your feelings and pursue your vision for the future about what you truly want so you can have a happy life at a healthy weight.

Reflection Questions

1. What inner roadblocks to your weight loss come from old patterns and outdated default rules you keep repeating?

2. When and how did these old patterns start?

3. What is one practical action goal you will apply to embrace living in the present moment more often?

How-To Guide

QUICK LIFE HACKS

Daily Gratitude Affirmation: Choose your future by adding this daily gratitude affirmation in the morning.

> *I am fortunate to be alive. I have a precious human life.*
> *I am not going to waste it.*

From *The Book of Joy* by the Dalai Lama, Desmond Tutu, and Douglas Abrams.[24]

Breathing: Each morning before you get up, allow yourself a moment to be in the present with this quick breathing exercise. Count to five as you inhale slowly and deeply and do the same as you exhale. Repeat this ten times to allow yourself to start the day calmly and with ease.

GUIDEBOOK EXERCISES

Exercise 12: Embrace the Present Moment
Exercise 13: Journal Daily

CHAPTER 14

Feeling Depleted

PROBLEM: Daily stress or lack of sleep leave me too tired for self-care.

PRINCIPLE: Manage stress and replenish yourself daily.

REMEMBER JEANETTE? Jeanette shared her desire to become healthy and fit and an example of healthy aging (see Chapter 8). Her two biggest challenges were stress from an overloaded work schedule coupled with being sleep-deprived. Yet, when she came to me, she simply anticipated making some changes in her diet. She was unaware of the roles that stress and sleep played in holding her back from a healthy lifestyle.

Jeanette told me that she had been eating dinner at 8:00 p.m. in her car at stop lights while driving from one client to another. She was often up until 1:30 a.m. writing follow-up emails from tutoring sessions. In short, she had almost no life outside of work and was too tired for self-care. What happened to Jeanette was remarkable. Together we created a plan that she implemented so she could stop work at 5:00 p.m. and get to bed on a regular schedule. These two changes became the foundation for her success in becoming fit, healthier, and losing weight.

Jeanette's problem of being too tired for self-care is more common than you may think and is why this chapter focuses on the problem of daily stress and lack of sleep. In this chapter, I'll show you how managing stress and adequate sleep can help you have the grit to change bad habits and replace them with good habits. We also talk about the different sources of stress, how they increase your appetite, and why they cause weight gain. We show you how to manage stress and replenish yourself daily as a Golden Key to having a happy life at a healthy weight.

Managing Daily Stress

Do you ever find yourself extra stressed and forget your good intentions to eat healthfully or go outdoors for a walk? There is a biological reason why stress stimulates hunger. One surprising fact is there are two different kinds of stress, and both increase your appetite but with differing results.

Acute stress happens when we encounter a sudden danger, like being chased by a saber toothed tiger. This danger requires a rapid fight-or-flight response. The part of our brain that responds to challenges like this is the limbic system. What happens that causes us to run from the saber-toothed tiger? The amygdala that governs basic emotions warns the hypothalamus, which then signals the rest of our body to take immediate action to fight or flee. With sudden danger, we experience an increased need for energy to respond to an immediate threat. To help meet the physical demands of acute stress, the hormone cortisol is released and stimulates hunger and eating that yields the quick energy required to fight or flee.

Chronic Stress

We no longer need to run from the saber toothed tiger. Instead, we face other types of small daily challenges that are chronic. The resulting chronic stressors cause our body to react differently. With chronic stress, our body also releases cortisol, which stimulates our appetite. At the same time, our body doesn't require more caloric energy to fight or flee. Instead, we merely fawn or freeze or these small bumps in the road go unnoticed. This increased hunger easily leads to eating more, storing more fat, and gaining weight.

Chronic disease is common. In the Stress in Americans Survey 2022 conducted by the American Psychological Association, 34 percent of adults reported that stress was "completely overwhelming most days." The majority, or 76 percent of adult respondents, said that "they have experienced health impacts due to stress in the prior month."[25]

The sources of daily chronic stress may not be recognized. In a February 2023 *Harvard Business Review* article, "The Hidden Toll of Microstress," by Rob Cross and Kane Dillon, the authors identified microstresses as the small, invisible, fleeting, stressors that seem like "small bumps in the road." These microstresses can be as small as taking fifteen minutes to help out a coworker. The authors noted that, "Microstress may be hard to spot individually, but cumulatively they pack an enormous punch."[26]

During interviews with high performers from thirty global companies, Cross and Dillon discovered that these high performers "were powder kegs of stress" and most of them didn't realize the extent of their struggles to keep up their work and personal lives. Neither did they realize that it was an accumulation of small events that were leaving them feeling overwhelmed.

These microstresses can accumulate from lack of self-care like not sleeping or getting enough physical activity. Lack of self-care adds to work or financial stresses, and together can lead to burn out and exhaustion. The authors pointed to how microstresses may affect weight. Cross and Dillon shared an example discussed by Lisa Feldman Barrett, distinguished professor of psychology at Northeastern University. Barret noted that in one study when a person experienced social stress within two hours of a meal, this stress added more than one hundred calories to the meal and could contribute to a weight gain of eleven pounds a year.

Overcoming Chronic Stress

Regular practices that elicit a relaxation response can keep microstressors from accumulating that leads to chronic stress. These regular practices include breathing exercises, meditation, and physical activity. As we've shown, chronic stress can lead to overeating, feeling controlled by food, and weight gain.

What can you do to overcome the tendency to overeat when stressed? A good place to start is with awareness that your body is trying to protect you. When your brain signals danger, one of your body's natural responses is increased appetite. I have shared our key signature tool with you, the Five Steps to Stop being Controlled by Food so you can choose a better response to food cravings, in Chapter 7. What else can you do as part of managing food cravings that come from chronic stress? With the intention of returning to a more relaxed place, consider what foods are calming and nurturing for you instead of turning to highly processed foods full of sugar, salt, and fat that can intensify food cravings. Make a list of foods that are nurturing and satisfying. My high coaching recommendation is to pay close attention to what you eat and combine choosing these nurturing foods with other activities that elicit a relaxation response like breathing exercises, meditation, and physical activity.

Oh, for a Good Night's Sleep

Could lack of sleep cause you to gain weight or prevent you from losing weight? One of my clients, Dan, who was struggling with obesity, said that he woke up tired each morning because he went to bed too late. When we did an assessment during one of our coaching sessions, he realized that going to sleep with the television on was interfering with getting enough sleep. Lack of a good night's sleep made it hard for him to focus on weight loss the next day. Once he solved this problem, he was able to wake up rested and start the day with the physical activity he needed to help him lose weight. What made the difference? He decided on a specific time to turn off the TV and go to bed.

Maybe you're like so many of the millions of Americans who are not getting enough sleep each night, and you decide you want to go to bed earlier and set a bedtime. What will your approach be? Do you believe you can learn this skill? Is it possible or impossible? This example illustrates the difference between two types of mindset—a fixed or growth mindset, which we talked about in Chapter 8.

To further illustrate these two different mindsets about sleep, let's say you want to feel more rested when you wake up in the morning. If you have a fixed mindset about sleep, you might say to yourself, "I'm a night owl. I've always been a night owl and I'll always be a night owl. Changing my bedtime is not going to work for me."

In contrast, the person with a growth mindset might say, "Now, usually I go to bed at midnight. Instead, I'm going to go to bed at 11:00 p.m. this week and see how it goes."

Lack of Sleep: The Sleep and Obesity Connection

How much sleep do adults need? Adults need seven or more hours of sleep a night according to the American Academy of Sleep Medicine and Sleep Research Society.[27] Sleep is important to physical, mental, and emotional health. Lack of sleep has several consequences, including higher rates of obesity for adults who don't get enough sleep. Short sleep duration is also linked to the development of type 2 diabetes, heart disease, and depression. The negative effects of lack of sleep touches nearly every area of life, including an impaired ability to think, learn, and recall.

Lack of sleep may contribute to weight gain and obesity. Interestingly, obesity rates have increased at the same time the hours of sleep a night have decreased.[28] Short sleep cycles are also associated with poor eating habits from meals and snacks, nighttime eating, and higher intake of fast foods, sugar, and fat. It also contributes to decreased energy and increased weight. How might sleep deprivation affect what we eat? Sleep-wake cycles influence circulating levels of appetite-regulating hormones, ghrelin, and leptin. Decreased sleep may disrupt appetite hormone regulation by increasing ghrelin, the hormone that stimulates the appetite, and by decreasing leptin, the hormone that signals a sense of fullness also called satiety. The disruption of these two hormones may lead to overeating. Extended hours of wakefulness create more time for eating. Many of the people I've worked with stay up late, snack at night, and then gain weight.

One-third of US adults don't get enough sleep. Work, social demands, and changes in technology have created a perfect storm of a lack of sleep, weight gain, and compromised physical and mental health. Getting enough sleep is one of the key components to success at having a happy life at a healthy weight.

How to Thrive: Manage Stress and Sleep to Replenish Yourself Daily

Arianna Huffington, author and founder of the *Huffington Post*, is a good example of someone who recovered from collapse because of sleep deprivation and burnout. According to Huffington and co-author Marina Khidekel, we need to change the way we work and end the delusion that burnout is the "price we must pay for success" as described in their book, *Your Time to Thrive, End Burnout, Increase Well-Being, and Unlock Your Full Potential With the New Science of Microsteps.*[29] These authors are dedicated to using tiny changes they call microsteps to create sustainable changes and improvements to health and happiness. Tiny changes can help us get a good night's sleep and better manage stress. We revealed and showed you how to consistently apply new habits in Chapter 12.

Getting Started

Where to begin? I recommend you take one tiny step at a time and take a stand for your health and well-being, starting with setting a regular bedtime. Why start small? Making a wholesale lifestyle change at once can create a boomerang effect and be counterproductive. Think of it this way: when you succeed with a tiny daily change, your confidence grows as you tackle each change that can compound to yield big results. The big payoff is that you can then live the life you want to live at the weight you want to be and look in the mirror and love who you see.

Chapter Summary

In this chapter, we introduced you to the whys and ways to leave behind fatigue caused by stress and lack of sleep so you can live the life you want to live—a happy life at a healthy weight. Tiny micro-changes are the best way to get started with new habits that can give you the energy to grow your confidence and succeed with weight loss that you can keep off and thrive in mind and body.

Companion Chapters for Exploration

Want more help with the problem that daily stress or lack of sleep leaves you too tired for self-care? Here's a recommended shortcut: pick one or more of the chapters below to read next that seem most relevant to you. (These are also listed on the ROADMAP chart in Chapter 4.)

EXPECTATIONS: I EXPECT QUICK RESULTS FROM DIETS AND CHANGING HABITS (CHAPTER 5)

I introduce the fallacy of expecting rapid and lasting results with a quick-fix diet that is temporary. Instead, use a comprehensive lifestyle approach that emphasizes making tiny changes that can make a big difference because they can be sustained for a lifetime (though not perfectly).

RUNNING ON EMPTY: I DON'T MAKE MYSELF A PRIORITY (CHAPTER 6)

This chapter demonstrates how to commit daily to declaring your worthiness and making yourself a priority. We share with you how to make time for yourself and schedule daily self-care and recognize that self-care is not selfish.

PEOPLE-PLEASING: I'M AFRAID TO DISAPPOINT OTHERS (CHAPTER 9)

People-pleasing causes us to trim our sails in life about what's possible because we are worried about what other people think and about winning their acceptance and approval instead of scheduling time for self-care. This chapter addresses what you can do about people-pleasing and what other people think.

LACK OF CONSISTENCY: I APPLY NEW HABITS, THEN THEY FALL BY THE WAYSIDE (CHAPTER 12)

Changing habits consistently is the Golden Key to solving the problem posed in this chapter: "I Apply New Habits, Then They Fall by the Wayside." You are given examples of how to build new habits with consistency and sustain new habits.

DISCONNECTED: I FORGET ABOUT MY BODY'S NEEDS (CHAPTER 16)

This chapter's purpose is to increase your sense of safety and ability to listen to your body's signals. As you align with your body's feedback, you may notice that it opens the door to trusting that your body's purpose is to protect you.

Reflection Questions

1. What problems do you have with stress and sleep?

2. How do problems impact your life?

3. What is one easy, tiny step you'll take this week bring to refresh yourself with managing stress or with sleep?

How-To Guide

QUICK LIFE HACK

Reset your circadian rhythm or improve your sleep cycle with a morning walk outdoors.

GUIDEBOOK EXERCISES

Exercise 14: Five Ways to Release Stress and Build Resilience

Resource 2: Tips for a Good Night Sleep

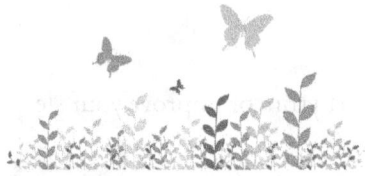

CHAPTER 15

Perfectionism Holds Me Back

PROBLEM: I beat myself up or give up if I don't carry out my aims perfectly.

PRINCIPLE: Let go of taking things personally. Choose progress not perfection.

Laurel's Example

One day when I was sitting in my office, I got a call from a lady named Laurel. She's a therapist in private practice and she works with people all day long and helps them get clear so they can live a stress-free and productive life. When she called me, she said: "I don't want another failed attempt at a diet, and I want to get my eating under control. I don't want to fall off the wagon and go back to old habits."

What usually happened was that after a few weeks of doing well, she'd start to snack again. Then, she would become so disappointed in herself that she continued snacking each afternoon when she wasn't even hungry for as long as a month until she finally stopped herself. She didn't want that old cycle to repeat itself yet again.

As a result of serving her clients all day long, the one thing Laura neglected was to allow herself self-care and nurture herself after work. She gave herself no break before she cared for her three children. Instead, Laurel ate candy, cookies, and crackers that she put out for her children to eat while she watched them play. When we looked at her life, that's when we found that she needed a break in the afternoon to nurture and take care of herself. She gave care to everyone else but herself. She was scared to give voice to her own need for self-care. After all, Laurel believed that as a wife, mom, and therapist she should have it all together and believed she should be and was trying to be perfect.

Things changed once Laurel allowed herself a break. She made time for a walk in between work and childcare to refresh her body and mind. It was then that she stopped her old snacking habit and had the energy to enjoy time with her kids.

Trying to be perfect, that's the thing that trips many of us up. Perfectionism first came into my life when I was a schoolgirl. My brother was always getting into trouble because of his grades. I didn't want to be that kind of kid, and I was terrified of not handing in a homework assignment on time. I had to do everything right. I would have rather died than miss homework deadlines. I was gripped with fear, and at the same time wanted my parents to be happy with my grades. I remember teachers writing on my report cards that, "Kathy worries too much about her schoolwork." To this day, perfectionism shows up in my life, now often as a fear of technology glitches, and I'm working on giving myself grace and compassion so I can move on instead of becoming like a deer in headlights when my screen freezes from internet instability, which is something that is out of my control.

How can we use the idea of "progress not perfection" to move forward to create a happy life at a healthy weight? First let's tackle the question of what perfectionism is. As Ella, one of the people I've helped, said to me, "Perfectionism means to me that if I don't carry out my aim perfectly, I beat myself up or I give up." It's so easy to beat ourselves up.

In this chapter, I'll show you three ways to transform perfectionism into progress by letting go of judgment and comparison, using curiosity to allow you to see things differently. The problem of wanting to be perfect is an obstacle to a happy life at a healthy weight for so many of us.

My highest coaching recommendation for you if you're looking for a happy life at a healthy weight is to allow yourself time for self-care in your busy life (especially if you have kids).

How else can you disrupt a habit of striving to be perfect? Let's start with awareness of what you are doing now. Notice symptoms like "black or white" and "all or nothing" thinking when they crop up. Start by asking yourself, "How do I usually approach the choices I make?"

Do you make choices by judging yourself or with curiosity? We begin with judging and then look at curiosity as the key to transformation.

Let's look at an example from the workplace. Consider a boss who feels the need to be right and sees members of his team as the problem because they are raising objections about an approach he wants to take on a project. He asks, "What's wrong with them?" He judges himself as right and other team members as wrong. You can meet a boss who is taking a "judger path" in the book *Change Your Questions, Change Your Life: 10 Powerful Tools for Life and Work* by Marilee Adams.[30] The judger seeks to assign fault by asking what's wrong with them and what's wrong with him; a path that leads to the "judger pit" in the book's Choice Map graphic.

As Adams's book points out, we're all recovering judgers. An alternative to judging that comes with perfectionism is to become curious and ask helpful questions described on a Choice Map as a "learner path." These questions include asking things like what do I want? What can I learn? And what are my choices?

Let's delve further into how the tendency to judge yourself plays out. One of the ways judging shows up can be comparison. As author and mentor Heather Dominick pointed out in her book, *Different*, three distinctive forms of comparison may be at play.[31]

1. Comparison to others: You might compare yourself to what other people believe or achieve. Maybe you know somebody who has lost ninety-five pounds, and you've lost much less weight. You might ask, "What's wrong with me for not losing as much weight as he or she did?"

2. Comparison to what others expect: A tell-tale sign of comparison and judging yourself based on what others expect of you is when you hear yourself using the word "should." Do you "should" on yourself by asking yourself, "I should do _____ (you fill in the blank)?"

For example, you may hear yourself saying, "I *should drink* at the party tonight because otherwise my friends will call me a party pooper." Using the word "should" often comes from fear of disapproval that is linked to perfectionism. Perfectionism and people-pleasing often go hand in hand as you strive to meet the expectations of others.

3. Comparison with past or future: You might compare your current behavior with what you expect from yourself compared with your past or future. You might say, "I need to lose thirty more pounds before my birthday in six months." These kinds of comparisons and expectations can make you feel terrible because you're trying to live up to expectations that aren't feasible and can leave you feeling frustrated and unworthy.

There is a way you can dissolve a web of disappointment that you can unknowingly weave for yourself. What can you do instead of judging and comparing yourself and feeling belittled? Since we are all recovering judgers, nobody escapes completely. Frequent grace and compassion can help lead you away from this frustration so you can come home to who you truly are. Instead of comparing and judging, you might ask, "How can I shift what I'm comparing myself to into an idea that's right for me—for my values and my healthy mind and body?"

Example: "If I can eat food in an amount that's right for me, maybe I won't lose as much as Susie, but I'll lose what's right for me."

My highest coaching recommendation is to look inside yourself and ask what you really want and what really matters to you. When we catch ourselves seeing things as all or nothing, we have a chance to transform these thoughts into a both/and choice using curiosity and by asking revealing questions. According to Diane Hamilton, researcher and author of the book *Cracking the Curiosity Code*,[32] curiosity is at the heart of success according to her interviews with successful people.

Also, based on examining research on the topic of curiosity, she concluded that curiosity makes us feel good. In fact, when curiosity is triggered, dopamine is released. That is, we get the same kind of feel-good boost from dopamine when we are curious as when we snack on sugary foods.

It's natural to feel curious. And as B. F. Skinner wrote: *No one asks how to motivate a baby. A baby naturally explores everything it can get at unless it's being restrained, and that's already been at work. And this tendency doesn't die out, it's wiped out.*[33]

Curiosity is an instinct that is fundamental to the human experience. Curiosity begins prior to experiencing childhood conditioning and social expectations. As Skinner's quote implies, things that can hold us back from being curious include things like fear, childhood conditioning and societal values.

In her book, Diane Hamilton concluded that curiosity is the driving force of motivation, based on her review of existing studies on curiosity. Curiosity is a more powerful motivator than wealth and can lead to landing a better job and living a happier life according to her many interviews with many successful people, including Steve Forbes.

How Curiosity Helps Cure Perfectionism

Curiosity can lead us to inquiry and discovery of three things that can loosen the hold that perfectionism can have on us:

Self-compassion: Empathy helps us forgive ourselves because we are human and we all make mistakes. We all are recovering judgers. At times, we might compare ourselves to what we "should" do and/or what others think.

Choices: Knowing that we have choices, we can choose a path that allows us to receive the good in our lives.

Good enough: We can let go of perfectionism by allowing that we are good enough just as we are.

Chapter Summary

How can you let go of all-or-nothing thinking and choose progress not perfection? This chapter is designed to help you choose self-compassion and love, allow yourself to feel that you are good enough just as you are, and let go of perfectionism. Judging and beating yourself up are symptoms of perfectionism and cause you to give up on cherished dreams. Curiosity, compassion, and self-acceptance can allow us to make progress instead of being paralyzed by fear of being a failure when we don't carry out our aims flawlessly.

Companion Chapters for Exploration

Want more help with the problem that you beat yourself up or give up if you don't carry out your aims perfectly? Here's a recommended shortcut: pick one or more of the chapters below to read next that seem most relevant to you. (These are also listed on the ROADMAP chart in Chapter 4.)

I recommend inquiring with curiosity and self-acceptance where you can instead of judging yourself and others as you explore these chapters.

SELF-SOOTHING: I USE FOOD AS RELIEF FOR MOOD OR STRESS (CHAPTER 7)

We see that Katie, introduced in Chapter 1, reached out for help because when she got angry, sad, and lonely, she "stuffed her face" with food. I helped her disrupt this old pattern with our signature process of Five Steps to Stop Being Controlled by Food.

PEOPLE-PLEASING: I'M AFRAID TO DISAPPOINT OTHERS (CHAPTER 9)

People-pleasing causes us to trim our sails in life about what's possible because we are worried about what other people think and about winning their acceptance and approval instead of scheduling time for self-care. I address what you can do about people-pleasing and placing importance on what other people think.

FEELING STUCK: I DON'T KNOW WHY I KEEP REPEATING OLD PATTERNS (CHAPTER 13)

It's far easier to repeat old patterns when we aren't present in the moment and are unconscious of the choices we are making. In this chapter, we share how to heal the past, embrace the present, and choose your future.

DISCONNECTED: I FORGET ABOUT MY BODY'S NEEDS (CHAPTER 16)

This chapter's purpose is to increase your sense of safety and ability to listen to your body's signals. As you align with your body's feedback, you may notice that it opens the door to trusting that your body's purpose is to protect you.

TUNED OUT: MY LIFESTYLE CHOICES ARE LARGELY UNCONSCIOUS (CHAPTER 19)

For many of us, lifestyle choices are largely unconscious, and that causes us to overeat and forget about self-care. We share essential advantages and aspects of making conscious choices, including paying attention while eating and slowing down enough to tell when we're full without overeating.

Reflection Questions

What about you? Here's your opportunity to reflect on how to let go of perfectionism.

1. What is a time when you used curiosity to stop judging yourself and asked, "How can I look at this differently?"

2. What does your good enough weight loss look like and feel like, so you won't beat yourself up over food or self-image?

3. What is your biggest takeaway from this chapter on how to let go of perfectionism and how will you use it?

How-To Guide

QUICK LIFE HACK

Stop, Think, Ask: How can I create a few minutes for self-nurturing that puts me in a good mood instead of feeling put-upon and judging myself and others?

GUIDEBOOK EXERCISE

Exercise 15: Become Aware of and Counter Self-Criticism

CHAPTER 16

Disconnected

PROBLEM: I forget about my body's needs. I eat quickly, while distracted, when full, and/or skip meals. I don't get enough sleep.

PRINCIPLE: Align your choices with what your body needs.

WHEN JUSTIN CALLED ME FOR HELP, he said, "I have a problem with my weight and what I eat. I'm eating the wrong things at the wrong times." He also said, "At thirty-eight years old, I have to walk with a cane because of a knee injury. I can't be the dad I want to be because of my weight. I skip meals during the day, avoid eating dinner with the family, and then I binge eat at night."

We assessed what was driving his choices that caused him to continue to gain weight. This process was like a mirror that showed where he was when he came to me and what was possible.

During more than a year that we worked together, he began making different choices. Most importantly, he stopped skipping meals during the day, ate dinner with the family, and stopped binge eating at night. Now his knee is better, so he doesn't need surgery, and he goes to spinning classes four times a week. He has lost one hundred pounds that he has kept off for more than a year.

It's easy to forget about your body's needs when you have a busy day. Then again, when aren't your days busy? This chapter's purpose is to increase your sense of safety and ability to listen to your body's signals. As you align with your body's signals, you may notice that it opens the door to trusting that your body's purpose is to protect you. You may also become aware that when you are responding to its signals, you are loving and respecting your body.

What Gets in the Way?

Why is it so tempting to ignore our body's needs in the throes of daily activity? When busy, we avoid paying attention when our body tells us it is hungry, tired, or overly stressed because:

- ✧ We are creatures of habit

- ✧ We want results but resist making the changes needed to achieve them

- ✧ Social expectations lead us to dieting and self-restriction

I learned a hard lesson after decades of dieting failure that I described in this book's Introduction. I discovered the need to align with my body's needs after years of trying to punish my body into becoming the body of my dreams as I obsessively swung between "feast and famine" eating while I went on and off diets. I ate quickly when distracted, and ate even when I was full to soothe myself. Then, I slowly began listening to my body's signals and began to nourish myself and grow healthier. That's how I learned the importance of connecting with my body's needs.

I discovered how to eat when I was hungry, take walks and meditate to relieve stress, eat mindfully, and get a good night's sleep as the foundation for losing weight and keeping it off. My aim with this chapter is to help you put this foundation in place for your successful weight loss journey that begins with healing your relationship with food.

Collaborating with Your Body

Next, let's delve into how to collaborate with your body instead of overthinking, punishing, or trying to control it as you ignore your body's signals. How can you pay attention to what your body is asking of you instead of shutting down or ignoring your body's signals that you are hungry, tired, or stressed?

Make it Simple to Align with Your Body's Needs

I recommend keeping it simple by aligning with what your body needs. Let's explore how to make self-care an act of love by responding positively to what your body is asking of you. A helpful next step is to stop torturing yourself by denying yourself the pleasure of eating with restrictive dieting. Instead, empower yourself to live the life you want to live—the opposite of forcing yourself into restrictive dieting.

How to Align with What Your Body Needs

Next, we'll explore how you can respond to your body's signals in a way that will make your self-care easier and help you create a happy life at a healthy weight. What does it mean to align your choices with what your body needs as one of the core principles of our program? What follows are three simple guidelines that will allow you to align with what your body needs instead of ignoring them:

1. Eat when you're hungry.
2. Rest, sleep, and refresh yourself when tired.
3. Relax when you're stressed.

Sounds simple, right? These practices form the foundation of a flexible support structure instead of adhering to a rigid diet of dos and don'ts that aren't sustainable.

These simple guidelines can transform your busy life using small steps that can add up to big results. Interested in testing this idea? Try these three guidelines for a week. Notice any differences you experience from applying these guidelines. Do you feel more satisfied, rested, and less stressed? The intention is for you to improve your quality of life and progress by building a shame-free relationship with food by using these guidelines.

1. EAT WHEN HUNGRY

Why address hunger? The reason to stop fighting hunger is that it's dangerous to ignore hunger pangs, and here's why. Your body's most pressing job is to ensure your survival by protecting you from starvation. If your brain detects that you're starving, your body will become more efficient with what little fuel it has being given to preserve your body weight—at all costs.

Our species has survived for the last 130,000 years because of our biology. Our body has a life-enhancing mechanism made up of a strong appetite-stimulating hormone, ghrelin, known as "the hunger hormone," that urges us to eat. This strong hormone is coupled with leptin, a weak appetite-suppressing hormone, that decreases appetite and urges us to stop eating when full.

You will eventually become grumpy and stop losing weight if you are consistently hungry and refuse to allow yourself to eat. This is a path that, at worst-case scenario, becomes anorexia nervosa and can lead to death. Eating when you're hungry is the number one guideline for success in creating a happy life at a healthy weight. If you discover nothing else from reading this book, please remember not to live life by going around hungry and grumpy.

Karen Carpenter's Story

Karen Carpenter and her brother Richard were well-known as the Carpenters, a commercially successful and acclaimed soft rock duo of the 1960s and 1970s. Karen was one of the most popular singers of her generation. She struggled for years with anorexia nervosa, a hidden eating disorder that led to weight loss. She weighed only eighty-nine pounds at the time of her death in 1983. She was only thirty-two years old when she died from heart failure as a complication of anorexia. Fortunately, her heartbreaking story raised awareness of anorexia as a serious health issue for the first time. Sadly, her concern about her looks on stage led to her eating disorder and eventual death.

Her story was first captured in the film *The Karen Carpenter Story*, a TV movie which aired in 1989. Most recently, interviews with Karen Carpenter offered fresh insights into her inner emotional life in the documentary *Starving to Perfection*, created by Randy Schmidt and released at the Santa Barbara International film festival in February 2023.

I was a big fan of the Carpenters and still listen to some of their memorable music to this day. This story of Karen Carpenter always reminds me of my friend Christy, a ballet dancer who died in her twenties from the complications of anorexia nervosa. She never talked about her struggle with food, and it was sad to lose such a beautiful and talented friend at such a young age.

Skipping Meals Contributes to Overeating

Skipping meals can also lead to being overly hungry and overeating. It may be tempting to skip meals to lose weight or because of long work hours. Unfortunately, skipping meals can backfire. Some clients like Justin skipped breakfast and lunch, and often dinner. Then he ate large amounts of food afterwards. Learning to eat regular meals instead of binge eating at night was one of the keys to Justin's success in losing one hundred pounds during our work together, as we mentioned earlier in this chapter.

Meal skipping also is associated with early death according to a recent study of more than 24,000 adults aged forty years and older by Y. Sun et al. published in the Academy of Nutrition and Dietetics.[34] In this study, adults who ate only one meal a day had an increased risk of mortality from all causes and cardiovascular mortality. Among the findings, skipping breakfast and lunch was also associated with increased mortality.

Eating Quickly

Excess and chronic stress make it easier to fall back into old habits and eat mindlessly. Stress also makes it more likely that you'll eat as fast as you can because you have other important things to take care of. Have you considered that eating quickly and while distracted may prevent your brain from having enough time to detect when you're full? Eating quickly may also cause you to overeat, gain weight, and feel even more stressed.

2. REST, SLEEP, OR REFRESH YOURSELF WHEN TIRED

Have you ever asked yourself, "Why am I so tired?" Feeling exhausted can become a way of life. Where does daily exhaustion start? Let's dig a little deeper than just blaming it on stress. Could you be a people-pleaser? Maybe you're so busy taking care of everyone else that there's no time for you. Do your needs almost always fall to the bottom of the list? If this sounds like you, it's time to make self-care a priority. Lack of self-care may be the cause of your exhaustion and may jeopardize your future, health, career, and relationships.

Instead, you can choose to invigorate yourself, feel younger, and have the energy to do things you haven't done in years and take care of those you love. Try these seven highly effective strategies to boost your energy. These energy-boosting life hacks can give you the vitality you desire when practiced daily.

A. Get Enough Sleep: If you wake up exhausted it may be time to develop better sleep habits so you'll wake up refreshed. Good sleep habits are simple. Try going to bed at the same time most evenings and avoid screen time for an hour before bed.

B. Get More Physical Activity: Regular physical activity can make you feel alive. Cardio exercise can re-invigorate you, lift your mood, and give you more stamina.

C. Drink More Fluids: Not drinking enough fluids is a common cause of fatigue, and it can be remedied by the simple act of drinking more water and other low-calorie fluids.

D. Eat Foods for Energy: Having the right balance of nutrients at meals and meal spacing can keep you from feeling tired. Too little protein at meals can make you hungry and tired a couple of hours after a meal.

E. Get Your Vitamins and Minerals: Many individuals, including those trying to lose weight, may be lacking key vitamins or minerals. Taking a multivitamin and mineral tablet daily can prevent fatigue from the lack of key nutrients you may be missing.

F. Calm Your Mind: If you feel frazzled and stressed much of the time, you may want to find five to fifteen minutes each day to calm your mind. Keep stress in check so it doesn't accumulate during the work week.

G. Relax and Have Fun: Take time to unwind each week to make you feel like a new person.

Medical conditions like diabetes also can cause you to feel tired. Be sure to check with a medical professional if fatigue persists after making these simple and easy lifestyle changes. When Stan first called me, he said, "I can't figure out why I'm tired all the time."

He said he woke up exhausted each morning and then couldn't muster the energy for self-care before he went to work. After we did an assessment, he decided to act. He decided to turn off the TV before bed. Instead of falling asleep while watching the news, he now wakes up refreshed and has the energy for morning exercise.

3. RELAX WHEN YOU'RE STRESSED

What can we do about daily chronic stress? The automatic response to stress is usually to soothe ourselves by overeating, drinking, or something else. Our body gives us an initial dopamine boost and a sense of relief for a few minutes. As noted in Chapter 7, according to Judson Brewer, Associate Professor of Medicine and Psychiatry at the University of Massachusetts Medical School, "We have conditioned ourselves to deal with stress in ways that ultimately perpetuate it rather than release us from it."

In summary, what we think helps to reduce our stress only makes it worse.

Regularly Practicing a Relaxation Response

What else can you do now to start practicing a relaxation response that can help you disrupt the cycle of daily chronic stress? Changing your breathing pattern can make a huge difference. You can change your thoughts, feelings, and mind when you change your breath. When you change your mind, you can change your life. Since stress can build day by day, effectively managing stress takes daily practice. Other ways to de-stress include taking a break with:

✧   Physical activity that you enjoy

✧   Meditation or just slow, deep breathing

✧   Yoga or T'ai Chi

✧   Enjoyable activities like collaging, painting, or woodworking

A well-practiced relaxation response can enhance your ability to step into the sweet spot of your life and have a happy life at a healthy weight with practices that bring you progress, confidence, and self-acceptance rather than shame, perfectionism, and burnout.

Chapter Summary

This chapter focused on aligning your choices and giving your body what it needs instead of succumbing to resistance to change and allowing yourself to give up on what you really want. The three guidelines revealed in this chapter on how to align with your body's needs are:

✧   Eat when you're hungry

✧   Rest, sleep, and refresh yourself when tired

✧   Relax when you're stressed

Companion Chapters for Exploration

Want more help with the problem that you forget about your body's needs? Here's a recommended shortcut: pick one or more of the chapters below to read next that seem most relevant to you. (These are also listed on the ROADMAP chart in Chapter 4.)

EXPECTATIONS: I EXPECT QUICK RESULTS FROM DIETS AND CHANGING HABITS (CHAPTER 5)

We introduce the fallacy of expecting rapid and lasting results with a temporary quick-fix diet. Instead, use a comprehensive lifestyle approach that emphasizes making tiny changes that can make a big difference because they can be sustained for a lifetime (though not perfectly).

RUNNING ON EMPTY: I DON'T MAKE MYSELF A PRIORITY (CHAPTER 6)

This chapter shows how to commit daily to declaring your worthiness and making yourself a priority. We share with you how to make time for yourself and schedule daily self-care and recognize that self-care is not selfish.

EMPTINESS: I USE FOOD/ALCOHOL AS RELIEF FOR MOOD OR STRESS (CHAPTER 7)

We see that Katie (who we introduced in Chapter 1) reached out for help because when she got angry, sad, and lonely she "stuffed her face" with food. I helped her disrupt this old pattern and consistently apply new habits with our signature process of Five Steps to Stop Being Controlled by Food.

FEELING DEPLETED: DAILY STRESS OR LACK OF SLEEP LEAVE ME TOO TIRED FOR SELF-CARE (CHAPTER 14)

In this chapter we introduce you to the whys and ways to leave behind fatigue caused by stress and lack of sleep so you can live the life you want to live—a happy life at a healthy weight.

TUNED OUT: MY LIFESTYLE CHOICES ARE LARGELY UNCONSCIOUS (CHAPTER 19)

For many of us, lifestyle choices are largely unconscious, and that causes us to overeat and forget about self-care. We share essential advantages and aspects of making conscious choices, including paying attention while we eat and slowing down enough so we can tell when we're full without overeating.

Reflection Questions

1. How do you respond when your body tells you it's hungry, tired, or stressed?

2. What stops you from aligning with your body's needs?

3. What will you do to align with your body's needs?

How-To Guide

QUICK LIFE HACK

Hunger Test

How can you tell if you're hungry?

Put your hands on your stomach. Think of a range of hunger. At level one you feel so hungry you'll faint. At ten you are as full as you've ever been, like after a huge Thanksgiving feast. Feel what's going on in your stomach. Do you have any hunger pangs right now? If your hunger is a four or below, it's time to eat.

GUIDEBOOK EXERCISES

Exercise 16: Changing the Way You Eat to Avoid Overeating and Excess Hunger

Exercise 14: Five Ways to Release Stress and Build Resilience

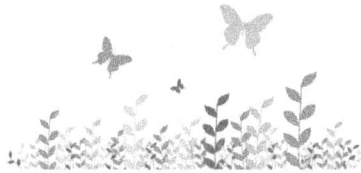

CHAPTER 17

Inspiring Action

PROBLEM: I start off strong, then I lose momentum.

PRINCIPLE: Recommit daily and inspire yourself to act on your intentions.

HOW CAN YOU ACCELERATE YOUR MOMENTUM once you discover your top motivators for a shame-free healthy relationship with food and live a happy life at a healthy weight?

How Doris Refueled Her Daily Commitment

When Doris first came to me, she said that she would sometimes eat a whole pumpkin pie in a day by herself, one sliver at a time. She told me that if she saw a tempting snack on TV, she'd immediately drive to the store, buy, and eat the snack. She said that she called me because she was twenty-five pounds overweight and because her blood sugar was close to the diabetic range. The most pressing thing in her life was to recover her health.

Doris had recently divorced, and she was midway through a successful career. She loved her job, but food was something she couldn't control. She wanted to make healthier food choices and lose weight. She had no energy. She wanted a different life. We did an assessment about why she overate. We clarified that her trigger was sitting in front of the TV. We homed in on her automatic response to snack on something sweet. She ate when she was bored. She knew something had to change.

Doris and I assessed her snacking patterns and came up with a plan. She vigorously implemented the plan. She overcame boredom by turning her weight loss project into a game. She got excited and inspired about competing with herself to get fit and lose weight. Then, she recommitted daily to her habit change goals. She challenged herself each morning to live her intentions. She continued to tell herself and me, "I'm not in competition with anyone else. I'm in competition with myself."

Doris became accountable by tracking her progress. She wrote down the calories she ate each day on her action goal sheet. She recommitted and renewed her motivation each day and challenged herself to do better than she'd done the day before. Her accountability also helped drive and renew her determination to be successful. She enthusiastically showed me her daily calories and progress on her action goals for the week each time we met.

Action and accountability fueled Doris's commitment. She stopped buying snack foods, trimmed her portions, and worked out more. She felt exhilarated when she walked every day at lunch. These walks proved to be a superb way for her to relax between work sessions. She worked out at a gym in the evening instead of sitting in front of the TV and snacking. She said, "I never thought I'd say this, but now I enjoy working out. Even on days when I don't feel like working out, I feel like I need to do something every day, even if it's just to take a short walk or lift weights."

After Doris lost twenty-five pounds, she continued to inspire herself and others by reminding herself and sharing her results. She said, "I have so much energy that sometimes in the evening I have to calm myself down because I'm so excited. I didn't want to do anything before, and now I'm ready to go."

Often, I hear people say that they don't understand why they lose their enthusiasm and motivation over time for a project like weight loss. Drive and motivation naturally wane over time and need to be renewed daily. In our busy lives, it's easy to get distracted by the many things that vie for our attention. As the popular quote says, often attributed to acclaimed and now deceased motivational speaker, Zig Ziglar, "People often say that motivation doesn't last. Well, neither does bathing, that's why we recommend it daily."

Inspiring Action and Consistency

Inspiration is the answer to the problem that when we start new habits, eventually our enthusiasm and drive drift away. The question is: How can we inspire ourselves consistently and recommit daily to act on our intended lifestyle choices that will help us lose weight? The answer is simple: spark consistency by inspiring ourselves every day. What works is to inspire ourselves to action. Take Doris's example: she generated her own enthusiasm rather than brow-beating herself into practicing new habits.

Actress Sheryl Lee Ralph was interviewed on *The Today Show* in 2022 after receiving an Emmy award for Best Supporting Actress from her role in the popular ABC TV comedy series, *Abbott Elementary*. She was asked about how she kept herself going all those years before her success as an actress and what advice had for the audience.

Ralph said she'd realized that it was up to her to cheer herself on and give herself hope daily, especially at her lowest moments. She explained, "I look in the mirror and I say, 'I love you.' I breathe in and out saying, 'In with the good and out with the bad.' I tell myself, 'We will get through this.'" Then she advised the audience, "Never give up on your dreams." She also asked, "Why be your own cheerleader?" She answered, "Because you are the only one who can truly lift yourself up."[35]

Three Ways to Inspire Yourself

How can you inspire yourself and cheer yourself on each day so that you act on your weekly Action Goals you've set for yourself?
Three ways to inspire yourself every day are to:

1. Uplift yourself. Use daily techniques that sustain you emotionally. Examples: Remind yourself why you are on this journey to a happy life at a healthy weight. Be your own cheerleader.

2. Start your day by doing something that brings you joy. For example, sing a song, practice your instrument, sketch an idea for your next painting, or work on your favorite puzzle.

3. Recommit each morning to refueling your weight loss drive and motivation.

Chapter Summary

The secret of weight loss success is to refuel your inspiration daily to spark commitment and consistency. Start your day by doing something joyful to inspire you to take a stand and empower yourself. Then refuel your weight loss drive by reviewing your action goals for the day out loud.

Companion Chapters for Exploration

Want more help with the problem that you start off strong, then lose momentum? Here's a recommended shortcut: pick one or more of the chapters below to read next that seem most relevant to you. (These are also listed on the ROADMAP chart in Chapter 4.)

EXPECTATIONS: I EXPECT QUICK RESULTS FROM DIETS AND CHANGING HABITS (CHAPTER 5)

We introduce the fallacy of expecting rapid and lasting results with a temporary quick-fix diet. Instead, use a comprehensive lifestyle approach that emphasizes making tiny changes that can make a big difference because they can be sustained for a lifetime (though not perfectly).

MINDSET: I DON'T BELIEVE I CAN SUCCEED (CHAPTER 8)

We explore how your mindset and beliefs from the past may interfere with weight loss, and how to cultivate a mindset shift that will help you master new habits.

MOTIVATION: I LOSE TRACK OF WHY WEIGHT LOSS MATTERS (CHAPTER 11)

This chapter emphasizes how easy it is to lose sight of your why—that is, why weight loss matters. Instead, we give you helpful ways to get and stay motivated during your weight loss journey. We also show you how to keep your reasons for losing weight in full sight. We ask you to envision the kind of person you want to become and change conflicting beliefs that can help you stay focused during your weight loss journey.

LACK OF CONSISTENCY: I APPLY NEW HABITS, THEN THEY FALL BY THE WAYSIDE (CHAPTER 12)

Changing habits consistently is the Golden Key to solving the problem posed in this chapter. We show how to build new habits with consistency and sustain them.

PERFECTIONISM HOLDS ME BACK: I BEAT MYSELF UP OR GIVE UP IF I DON'T CARRY OUT MY AIMS PERFECTLY (CHAPTER 15)

Judging and beating yourself up are symptoms of perfectionism and cause you to give up on cherished dreams. Curiosity, compassion, and self-acceptance can allow us to make progress instead of being paralyzed by fear of being a failure when we don't carry out our aims flawlessly.

Reflection Question

What is one thing you can do or say to yourself every day to inspire yourself to act on your good intentions?

How-To Guide

QUICK LIFE HACK

Read from an inspiring book, listen to a podcast, or watch a film for inspiration. Examples are: *The Book of Joy*, a podcast by Tara Brach, or watch a film like *The Power of the Heart*.

GUIDEBOOK EXERCISES

Exercise 17: Inspired Consistency

Exercise 14: Five Ways to Release Stress and Build Resilience

Resource 1: ROADMAP Daily Action Plan

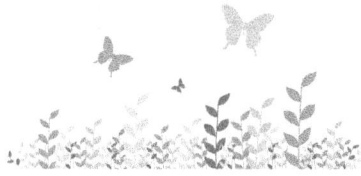

CHAPTER 18

Building Confidence

PROBLEM: I'm afraid of failing or succeeding at weight loss.

PRINCIPLE: I focus on changing the things I can change and accepting the things I cannot change.

Jennifer's Fear of Being Seen at Her New Weight

Jennifer gave a holiday party and went to a few holiday parties the year after the end of the pandemic. During the pandemic, she had lost forty-five pounds. She had worked with me for eight months and was making good progress with her weight loss. Suddenly, she hit a brick wall. Why? What surprised Jennifer was that that holiday season was the first time that friends and family had seen her and had commented on her new weight. These comments shook her to the core. She felt afraid. She feared it might not be safe to be at her new weight because it garnered unwanted attention and even snarky comments. She experienced resistance to moving forward with her desire to lose more weight because of this fear. Then, Jennifer felt a cascade of emotions.

She had reached a turning point and asked herself, "Am I going to stop the program to lose weight?"

She questioned whether the program was working for her. Why had she suddenly stopped losing weight even though she was eating the same as before and was doing the same activities?

Nothing had changed, and yet everything had changed for Jennifer. She dug deep and assessed what was going on because she had hit a point where she thought, "I'm not going to do this anymore. I don't think this program is working for me. I just don't think I'm going to be able to be successful at this." She told me, "I don't do very well when I'm not successful. I always pride myself in following through when I take on something."

Jennifer's husband encouraged her to sit with the question of whether to continue her weight loss journey. Given time for reflection, she realized that she didn't want to go back to the old habits, and ways of doing things. Jennifer chose to reframe her challenge and see things differently. Then, she decided to continue moving forward. After a couple of months of considering what to do, she felt much better. Then, things began moving in the right direction. She's back on track with losing weight.

Jennifer had lost confidence in her ability to do this work because of a setback during the holidays. It took her three months to regain her bearings after discovering that success was a little scary and had made her feel unsafe. Previously, her weight had protected her against unwanted attention. By allowing and exploring her feelings, Jennifer found a way to feel safe at a new weight and accept reactions to her weight change from the people she knew.

Roadblocks to Change

Many of us can recall a time when we started our journey to building new habits and how our confidence increased as we experienced progress. Then, BAM! Seemingly out of nowhere, we experienced obstacles, began to feel lost, and experienced resistance to continuing our journey. Just like Jennifer, we can struggle with a fear that can become a roadblock to progress.

Setbacks to change can present themselves in many forms. We avoid and resist what we know we need to do for the reason that we want to avoid the feelings of anxiety and defenselessness when we feel unsafe. We begin questioning ourselves and ask questions like, "What if I fail?" Or sometimes even scarier, we may ask, "What if I succeed?" Then, we either choose to act and use self-care to grow our confidence and succeed or we walk away in defeat. We may revert to old patterns of coping and feel shame and judge ourselves and others. Oddly, these old familiar patterns can feel like the right choice because they once worked well for us as far back as in childhood. Falsely, old patterns may feel like the safest choice.

The "Start Where You Are" chart below depicts the choice point that results from situations like Jennifer's that bring up fear and doubt. This can derail our intentions for our new vision of the future or become an opportunity to give ourselves grace and compassion and use grit and perseverance to re-ignite our commitment to our new vision of the future. The "Start Where You Are" chart below, adapted from the *Resistance to Resilience Chart* in the book *Different* by Heather Dominick, is designed for use when we are at a crossroads between giving up and moving forward.

Start Where You Are

Emotional state: Avoidance or Resistance

Fear, anxiety

↓

I feel unsafe

↓

I feel unable

↓

Stop

Old Habit   ⟵   Choice Point   ⟶   New Habit

Old coping pattern   ⟵   ⟶   Grace

Shame   ⟵   ⟶   Grit

Judgement   ⟵   ⟶   Resilience

Opportunity to Choose:
To Be Present
Practice intentions daily and build confidence

Fear as a Roadblock to Change

Why does fear cause us to avoid change? Recently, Leora called me for help because she wanted to lose weight. Here's what she told me. She was on a medication in her thirties that had a side effect of weight gain. At first, she felt good about her new weight because she got more respect than when she was younger, thinner, and wore a tiny dress size. She had adopted the belief that more weight meant greater respect.

We discovered that the fear of getting less respect from others if she lost weight had become a roadblock to losing and keeping it off. Now in her sixties, Leora is in the process of letting go of the hidden belief that she will get more respect by carrying extra weight. Instead, she now understands that the extra weight contributes to her back and knee pain. She places greater value on her health, her wish to be pain-free, and her mobility. Her health is a leading value that drives her commitment to lose weight and keep it off.

Fear is an inner roadblock that can cause us to act in ways that can become an obstacle. Symptoms of a fear of success can show up when we avoid doing what we know we need to do to get us where we want to be. Symptoms that get in our way can show up when we make excuses, complain, and blame ourselves or others.

How Brent Turned Fear of Success and Blame into Accelerated Weight Loss

When Brent first came to me, he told me he was afraid that he couldn't lose weight because his wife made such delicious desserts that were always around the house. He blamed her for his overeating. After we did an assessment, Brent understood that this blame wasn't helping. When he realized his weight gain was not his wife's fault, he made a different choice and acted on his new awareness. He advocated for himself by asking her to limit making desserts because, as he told her, sweets triggered him to lose control and overeat like an alcoholic with booze. Each weekend when they discussed meals for the week, he thanked her for her support during the past week. He also asked her again not to make desserts and serve fruit instead. By advocating for himself and repeatedly asking for help, Brent accelerated his weight loss.

ACT Change Process

How can you let go of old unhelpful habits, replace them with new ones, and take the journey to a shame-free, healthy relationship with food and a happy life at a healthy weight? Let's dive into a framework for the change process. The change process I use is a three-step process for change that starts with **awareness**. The awareness step has three parts that include:

✦ Clarifying your current mindset and beliefs

✦ Assessing and acknowledging what's working and not working

✦ Uncovering what it is you truly want

The second step, **creative discovery**, takes you further to allow, accept, and appreciate your feelings and what you value most. Lastly, the **transformation** step is designed to focus your effort on what you want to change with a new set of options and choices to help you act and master new habits.

Figure 4. ACT Change Process

Awareness	Become aware of your mindset, patterns, and what you truly want.
Creative Discovery	Allow, accept, and appreciate your feelings and what you value most.
Transformation	Turn what's not working into options for better lifestyle choices. Expand your vision. Let go of feelings and patterns that no longer apply to you Act on your true wishes.

Adapted from *Different* by Heather Dominick

Changing Your Response to Events

Another take on how to create what you truly want comes from Jack Canfield, a multiple *New York Times* best-selling author of, *The Success Principles, How to Get from Where You Are to Where You Want to Be.*[36] In his book, Canfield recommends where to focus your attention to successfully make changes in your life. According to Canfield, the only way you can influence life's outcomes is by changing your response to what happens to you. He wrote, "If you don't like your outcomes, change your response."

Figure 5.

Canfield's formula to influence outcomes is:

Event + Response = Outcome

Jack Decided Not to Throw His Weight Around:

When Jack Canfield recently interviewed me about this

book, he revealed how he had dealt with his underlying fear and experience with his weight. Two defining events that had happened earlier in his life affected his weight. Jack told me:

> I had a gallbladder operation about thirty years ago and I lost a lot of weight as a result of the surgery. I just didn't feel like eating. And I got really thin and started to feel really uncomfortable. And I looked at that discomfort and it was because I didn't have any weight to throw around.
>
> The idea was that you should throw your weight around that I learned when I grew up in an all-boys military school, which was very macho, and I played football and all that stuff. I had a coach who wanted me to be a tackle instead of an end. He wanted to fatten me up so I'd be a big lineman. And I realized, wow, this is part of why I don't want to lose weight because I'm afraid I won't feel substantial. And I was able to deal with that. But I mean, it's interesting how many things are unconscious that you don't even know are there.[37]

Weight problems and associated health conditions are a good example of how we can change our response to an event. In the United States and other industrialized countries, the environment promotes weight gain. Obesity that results from weight gain can lead to a number of chronic diseases. Environmental changes in the last fifty years have led to a marked increase in body weight, so that nearly 75 percent of Americans are now overweight or obese. What are the implications for weight loss? Having a weight issue isn't your fault. It's a default response to an environment that encourages us to overeat cheap, plentiful, and highly processed food products and be sedentary.

What can you do? You can change your response to the environment, starting with what foods you buy. You don't have to cave in with an automatic default response from everyday exposure to convenient, ultra-processed foods. Overeating foods that are high in sugar, saturated fat, and salt can lead to weight gain and chronic health conditions like diabetes, high blood pressure, and heart disease. Given your lifestyle, what things can you change to have a happy life at a healthy weight?

How Can You Overcome Fear?

We all have fears and aspirations. Fear can make it difficult to overcome inertia and move forward with what we truly want. What is the antidote to fear? My highest coaching recommendation is to choose love over fear, starting with self-compassion. As US Surgeon General Vivek Murthy wrote: "The world is locked in a battle between fear and love. Choose love always. It's the world's oldest medicine."[38]

A second way to overcome fear is to discover how to build confidence and a determination to succeed.

How to Increase Your Confidence

Sandy is a physical therapist who has been helping other people during a long, successful career. During the day, she takes great care of other people. Then she goes home and wants to do nothing. When she first called my office, she told me that she was frustrated with wanting to eat food that's not healthy and eat for every emotion and occasion. She said that she had an addictive personality. Her extra weight affected her self-esteem, and she didn't feel good about herself. She recognized the connection between her relationship with food and her mental health. She wanted to lose weight and reinvent herself.

Sandy wished she could commit to putting in the effort and follow-through so she could lose weight and keep it off. Yet she had fears about not being able to do the work that would enable her to succeed. She was afraid to fail. She told me that her issues related to weight had contributed to her divorce. She started with a regular workout routine with a trainer and having a smoothie for breakfast. Yet, fear of failure kept her stuck. She lacked the confidence to believe she could succeed because of her past. She'd beat herself up for not allowing herself to take other small steps to help her build confidence in herself.

Then one day a few weeks ago, she was diagnosed with diabetes, and that brought to her attention the fact that her health was at stake. She began to clearly see that her dreams for the future could easily slip away if she ignored this wake-up call. She is paying attention now, especially to her food choices, because she wants to travel to all the national parks by RV and be here to see her grandchildren grow up.

I've helped hundreds of adults with their weight and their health. I've noticed in these last dozen years that when clients repeatedly act on their good intentions, they do better and better and increase their confidence in losing weight. These repeated actions are akin to what it takes to build the muscle strength that becomes increased motivation to keep going. Simply put, they acted with greater confidence and were more willing to keep doing the helpful behaviors that moved them toward a desired outcome.

How Justin Built His Confidence to Easily Receive Compliments

Justin became afraid and unsettled when he thought about what would happen when people noticed and commented that he had lost one hundred pounds while working with me. He hadn't seen many of his friends and colleagues since the beginning of the pandemic. He feared being judged and not responding well to comments about his weight. Justin and I worked together and created a response to such comments that turned his fear into confidence. His new response to compliments about his weight was simply to say, "Thank you." Then, he guided the conversation along in a helpful direction. This planned response allowed Justin to build his confidence and easily receive compliments about his new weight.

Confidence is something I have grappled with for years. Naturally, I was fascinated when I attended a women's business conference, and keynote speakers Katty Kay and Claire Shipman described their study of women and confidence as journalists and co-authors of *The Confidence Code: The Science and Art of Self Assurance, What Every Woman Should Know.* They examined what makes for confidence and lack of confidence in women on topics from sports and the military to politics and neuroscience. Kay and Shipman concluded that stewing and ruminating hold women back more often than men and offered sound advice that women: "Do more. Think Less" to grow their confidence. The authors prescribed a combination of preparation and practice to put women in a "zone of confidence." Most importantly, they concluded that:

> If you choose not to act, you have little chance of success. What's more, when you choose to act, you're able to succeed more frequently than you think. How often in life do we avoid doing something because we think we will fail? Is failure really worse than doing nothing? And how often might we actually have triumphed if we had just decided to give it a try?[39]

Kay and Shipman's findings are exactly on point. Acting on your own behalf significantly increases your chance for successful weight loss in contrast to doing nothing. It takes confidence, determination, and focus to go the distance and make lifestyle changes to build a healthy relationship with food for a happy life at a healthy weight.

Chapter Summary

With this chapter, I team up with you to create a supportive container designed to help you summon the courage to change the things you can change and embark on a change process to overcome patterns, including the fear that holds you back. This chapter is designed to help you grow your confidence in a way that aligns with your values to live a happy life at a healthy weight.

Companion Chapters for Exploration

Want more help with the problem you're afraid of failing or succeeding at weight loss? Here's a recommended shortcut: pick one or more of the chapters below to read next that seem most relevant to you. (These are also listed on the ROADMAP chart in Chapter 4.)

ROOTS OF SHAME (CHAPTER 1)

This chapter addresses the fear of letting go of childhood survival mechanisms that once served us well and that can become underlying shame that leads to overeating.

SELF-SOOTHING: I USE FOOD/ALCOHOL AS RELIEF FOR MOOD OR STRESS (CHAPTER 7)

We see that Katie, who we introduced in Chapter 1, reached out for help because when she got angry, sad, and lonely she "stuffed her face" with food. I helped her disrupt this old pattern and consistently apply new habits with our signature process of Five Steps to Stop Being Controlled by Food.

MINDSET: I DON'T BELIEVE I CAN SUCCEED (CHAPTER 8)

We explore how your mindset and beliefs from the past may interfere with weight loss, and how to cultivate a mindset shift that will help you master new habits.

FEELING STUCK: I DON'T KNOW WHY I KEEP REPEATING OLD PATTERNS (CHAPTER 13)

It's far easier to repeat old patterns when we aren't present in the moment and are unconscious of the choices we are making. This chapter shares how to heal the past, embrace the present, and choose your future.

TUNED OUT: MY LIFESTYLE CHOICES ARE LARGELY UNCONSCIOUS (CHAPTER 19)

For many of us, lifestyle choices are largely unconscious, and that causes us to overeat and forget about self-care. We share essential advantages and aspects of making conscious choices, including paying attention while while eating and slowing down so we can tell when we're full without overeating.

Reflection Question

To deepen your understanding of how fear may hold you back for your desired vision of your weight loss success, set aside a few minutes to reflect on and write your responses to this question:

What fears do you have about your ability to lose weight and keep it off? Include fear or failure or fear of success and consider the examples in this chapter.

How-To Guide

QUICK LIFE HACK

What is one thing that is within your power to change to help you lose weight?

GUIDEBOOK EXERCISE

Exercise 18: ACT Change Process in Action

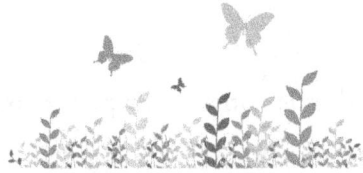

CHAPTER 19

Tuned Out

PROBLEM: My lifestyle choices and eating are largely unconscious.

PRINCIPLE: Be aware of and make lifestyle choices consciously.

JOY IS A DOCTOR AND A WIDOW who doesn't have children. She works all day, and, on her way home, she stops by a fast food restaurant and picks up a burger and fries for dinner. She eats in the car in the parking lot. She eats as fast as she can because she wants to get dinner over with and go home. Yet she has little to look forward to except to call her ailing mother.

When Joy called me for help, the first thing she said was that she was tired of gaining weight. I did an assessment and noticed that Joy had few pleasures in life. We created a plan. She acted on this plan so that she could enjoy eating again.

She created a special dinner for herself at home. She smiled as she bought flowers for herself for the first time in a long time, and later smiled again as she put them in a vase. She cleared the table of papers and magazines that had piled up over the months and spread a decorative and clean tablecloth over the table. She turned on music that she loved and cooked her favorite foods. She sat down, relaxed, and ate dinner slowly, taking in the aromas, textures, and flavors as she savored her food. This was how Joy created an enjoyable and mindful eating experience for herself.

What's the secret to making more intentional lifestyle choices? During my own journey of building a healthy relationship with food, here's how I discovered ways to make conscious lifestyle choices. One thing that especially helped was meditation. I started meditating in my twenties to calm myself and feel less stressed. Now I realize that being able to create more equanimity in my life helped me to make changes that I wanted to make so I could live in my sweet spot: healthier in mind, my body at the weight I wanted to be, and the ability to look in the mirror and love who I see. I changed my life, and I'm confident you can change your life, too.

This chapter addresses one of the most frequent problems that gets in the way of having a happy life at a healthy weight. The problem is that we make choices unconsciously.

Unconscious and Conscious Choices

Of course, not every decision we make needs to be conscious. We conserve mental energy by building skills and routines, like how to brush our teeth, that don't require us to be fully conscious, using our undivided attention. Yet, some of our unconscious patterns may no longer be helpful and instead may be inner roadblocks to what we truly want.

What are your unconscious lifestyle choices that have become obstacles? It may help to notice the lurking symptoms of unconscious choices. Do you notice that you have a tendency to:

✧ Avoid doing what you know you need to do

⟡   Worry about what other people think

⟡   Eat mindlessly while distracted

If so, there's likely a gap between your intentions and behaviors if you're stuck in old patterns. What unconscious choices do you want to address to accelerate your weight loss momentum?

Conscious Choices

When making lifestyle changes, we can make progress when we purposefully disrupt old routines that are no longer helpful. Then we can replace old patterns with new habits by making conscious choices. Healing starts with awareness. As Haruki Murakami, a famous Japanese author, wrote: "Pain is inevitable. Suffering is optional."[40]

It's our choice about whether to become aware of what we've doing in the moment so we can make better lifestyle choices.

When you become aware of what you feel and what you truly want, you'll be more likely to make a conscious choice for yourself. How can you make these conscious lifestyle choices?

1. Discover what you truly want that may be different from what others want or expect.

2. Allow yourself to feel and accept your feelings.

3. Create your own rules rather than following social expectations, especially those that apply to body image and dieting.

4. Become aware of what you're doing in the moment while you're eating instead of being distracted by other activities.

5. Tap into your innate self-compassion by accepting that mistakes are what help us grow.

Here are three specific steps to free yourself and make conscious lifestyle choices more often:

✧   Start where you are by accepting the unwanted parts of yourself to create compassion for yourself and others.

✧   Discover the Myth of Multitasking.

✧   Slow down when you eat: experience the tastes and textures. Eat more mindfully instead of eating quickly to get it over with.

Self-Compassion

Self-acceptance and self-compassion are necessary to make the change process outlined in Chapter 18 work, so that we can live a happy life at a healthy weight. Why? It takes courage to look the unwanted parts within us in the eye and accept them. In her remarkable book, *Start Where You Are, A Guide to Compassionate Living*, Pema Chodron, a Tibetan Buddhist nun, explained that we are most in need of compassion for ourselves when we encounter the parts of ourselves that are unwanted and rejected. Chodron, a plain spoken, down-to-earth divorced mother and grandmother from Kansas, became a Tibetan Buddhist nun after her husband left her for another woman. According to Chodron, we suffer when we encounter unwanted parts within and then give up on ourselves. She wrote that, as a result, "We keep missing the moment we're in. Yet, if we can experience the moment we're in, we discover that it is unique, precious, and completely fresh."[41]

I loved that Chodron recommended to "start where you are" as the key to self-acceptance and self-compassion. I was relieved to hear her message that as we allow all parts of ourselves in, we can relax and open, get to know our personal pain, and have a fresh start by being present in the moment.

Another champion of compassion, Tara Brach, author and teacher of mindfulness and meditation, described a process for cultivating compassion in her book *Radical Compassion, Learning to Love Yourself and Your World with the Practice of RAIN*. As Brach wrote, this is a process designed to help you access your naturally compassionate nature and "live true to yourself and actively care for others."[42]

I learned a version of this tool from from leadership mentor and author Heather Dominick, has helped me manage emotions such as anger and shame and reach a better understanding and a more compassionate acceptance of situations, others, and myself.

A basic outline of the RAIN process is to:

R = Recognize a situation that triggers stress within you
A = Allow and feel the emotions that surface from this stress
I = Investigate the situation with curiosity and kind attention
N = Nurture yourself with self-care to feel loved and safe

What I've discovered about self-compassion from these wise and courageous women is that I no longer need to second guess and beat myself up or make myself wrong. I can look at myself and others through the lens of understanding and loving kindness.

Multitasking

Do you often get distracted while eating and find that you're unaware of what you're eating? One of my clients referred to this distracted eating as "blackout eating." Maybe you eat while watching TV or while on another device. Distractions like these often lead to overeating, weight gain, and frustration.

As Sharon Salzberg shared in her article, "The Myth of Multitasking," our brain can focus only on one thing at a time.[43] Salzberg noted that what happens when we attempt to multi-task is that we shift attention between tasks and take in information sequentially. This means that we can't concentrate on two or more things at once. According to Salzberg, this shift back and forth wastes time and lowers the quality of what we do. I agree and believe that multi-tasking while eating makes us largely unconscious of our eating experience. Then we often eat more.

Enjoying Mindful Eating

Paying attention and staying in the present when we are eating is a simple way to enjoy our food and recognize when we're no longer hungry. How can you enjoy the moment you are in and enjoy mindful eating?

Eating and the Brain

Our human brain takes fifteen minutes to register the food we've eaten and then signal satiety (when we are full). When we eat quickly, our brain often doesn't have enough time to tell us when we're getting full. Then we tend to overeat. Distracted eating can cause us to feel unsatisfied, overeat, and gain weight. There's actually a biological reason for you to slow down and enjoy eating mindfully.

Brandon's Story

When Brandon called for help, he told me his story. He was creating the life he wanted to live, but there was something he couldn't control. He wanted to eat healthier and lose weight, but it was difficult. He said that nothing was working.

We did an assessment and found out that he had an old habit of piling too much food on his plate without thinking. Then he felt guilty as he thought about his grandmother criticizing him and saying, "Your eyes are bigger than your stomach." The result was that Brandon ate everything on his plate just as fast as he could, and it was too fast for him to recognize when he was full and stop eating.

We created a plan, and Brandon consistently implemented his plan to slow down and mindfully enjoy his dinner and put less food on his plate. As a result, he ate less and lost weight. He had kicked the habit of overeating. Eating mindfully by making conscious choices became a powerful tool for Brandon to enjoy eating again, eat less, and lose weight that he could keep off.

Mindful eating is a powerful way to switch from a stress response to a relaxation response, especially when coupled with regular meditation and other relaxation techniques.

Chapter Summary

With this chapter, we've shared essential aspects of making conscious choices and disrupting old patterns so you can take a stand, empower yourself, and actively choose to live in your sweet spot at the weight you want to be and look in the mirror and love who you see.

Companion Chapters for Exploration

Want more help with the problem that your lifestyle choices are largely unconscious? Here's a recommended shortcut: pick one or more of the chapters below to read next that seem most relevant to you. (These are also listed on the ROADMAP chart in Chapter 4.)

If you've found this chapter helpful, I recommend you dive into these other chapters to further explore how to make conscious choices:

SELF-SOOTHING: I USE FOOD/ALCOHOL AS RELIEF FOR MOOD OR STRESS (CHAPTER 7)

We see that Katie, who we introduced in Chapter 1, reached out for help because when she got angry, sad, and lonely, she "stuffed her face" with food. I helped her disrupt this old pattern and consistently apply new habits with our signature process of Five Steps to Stop Being Controlled by Food.

PEOPLE-PLEASING: I'M AFRAID TO DISAPPOINT OTHERS (CHAPTER 9)

People-pleasing causes us to trim our sails in life about what's possible because we are worried about what other people think and about winning their acceptance and approval instead of scheduling time for self-care. This chapter addresses what you can do about people-pleasing and what other people think.

LACK OF CONSISTENCY: I APPLY NEW HABITS, THEN THEY FALL BY THE WAYSIDE (CHAPTER 12):

Changing habits consistently is the Golden Key to solving the problem posed in this chapter, "I Apply New Habits, Then They Fall by the Wayside." I show how to build new habits with consistency and sustain new habits.

FEELING STUCK: I DON'T KNOW WHY I KEEP REPEATING OLD PATTERNS: (CHAPTER 13)

It's far easier to repeat old patterns when we aren't present in the moment and are unconscious of the choices we are making. This chapter shares how to heal the past, embrace the present, and choose your future.

BUILDING CONFIDENCE: I'M AFRAID OF FAILING OR SUCCEEDING AT WEIGHT LOSS (CHAPTER 18):

Are you afraid when you think about losing weight? In this chapter, I focus on how fear can easily lead to self-sabotage and sidetrack you from your intentions. Instead, I recommend that you focus on the things you can change as you make lifestyle choices that will support you on your weight loss journey. Then I offer ways to choose your future with a change process and ways you can choose your response to events for a better outcome.

Reflection Questions

1. What keeps you from conscious lifestyle choices, including mindfully eating?

2. How can you be more present and make conscious choices like enjoying eating more mindfully?

3. What are you willing to commit to this week to make a conscious lifestyle choice?

How-To Guide

QUICK LIFE HACK

An easy way to make better choices is to slow down while you eat and be in the present moment. If you multitask when you eat, pick a meal and allow yourself to slow down and savor your food without plugging into digital devices. Instead, notice the flavors, textures, and colors.

GUIDEBOOK EXERCISES

Exercise 19: On Cultivating Compassion
Exercise 20: Eating Mindfully

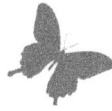

PART 3
Lifestyle Guide for a Happy Life at a Healthy Weight

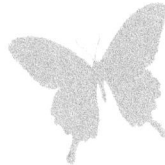

Understanding and applying the practical strategies
and skills for building sustainable change

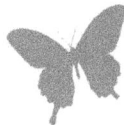

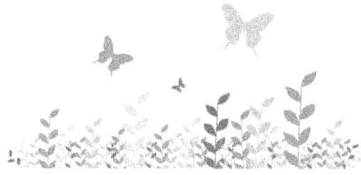

CHAPTER 20

Your Guide to Eating and Physical Activity

REMEMBER JUSTIN FROM CHAPTER 16? From an assessment we completed at the beginning of his program, we discovered that he had gained weight because he skipped meals during the day and binged after dinner at night. He had steadily gained weight and was walking with a cane because of a knee injury. During the program and partnership, he lost one hundred pounds and has kept it off for two years. He is off all medications, including medication for high blood pressure. How did he lose weight? He lost weight by following our comprehensive lifestyle change approach, most significantly by eating regular meals and taking a spinning class regularly.

With my comprehensive lifestyle change approach, I focus on habit changes that fit your lifestyle instead of a cookie cutter diet. This approach is designed to help you build a shame-free healthy relationship with food, lose weight, and keep it off for a happy life at a healthy weight. How it works is that I help you break free from food triggers and lifestyle choices that cause overeating.

Start by focusing on the power of healing the connection between food and shame and healing this connection. The program is further designed for you to remove inner roadblocks to weight loss and nurture yourself with conscious food choices, physical activity, and healthier lifestyle choices. Some of these lifestyle choices have already been covered in Part 2, for example, Chapter 14: Feeling Depleted, Daily stress or lack of sleep leave me too tired for self-care. This chapter gives you the tools to select your customized Healthy Eating and Physical Activity Plans.

Why Select a Customized Healthy Eating Plan?

By eating selectively and mindfully, you can build a healthy relationship with food while enjoying the foods you love. This lifestyle change starts by asking you to choose a healthy eating pattern that you can sustain and that includes your favorite foods if your goal is to shed excess weight and keep it off. Whichever plan you pick, you'll want to "be selective" about what and how much you eat to lose weight.

You'll be able to lose weight by selectively eating smaller amounts of higher-calorie foods and having having them less frequently. For example, if you love chocolate, consider eating a small amount of your favorite chocolate every day and/or save room for a rich chocolate dessert on special occasions. I love chocolate and freely admit that I eat at least one or two squares of dark chocolate daily. Some clients have said that they can't eat just a little of their favorite foods. If this sounds like you, you may want to save favorite treats for "special occasions" instead of eating them daily.

Sweet Life Wellness weight loss program offers a choice of three healthy eating plans. Why not just one food plan? Because you're more likely to succeed with a plan that is geared to your lifestyle and food preferences. Discover more about these plans in this section and more details in the How-To Guide for this chapter.

The first of these options is the *Sweet Life Wellness* Personalized Food Plan that you'll devise by looking at and making changes within your current eating pattern. If you prefer a more structured approach and want to adopt a heart-healthy eating pattern, consider choosing the Mediterranean dietary pattern or the DASH food plan. Each of these food plans is briefly described below.

Three Healthy Eating Plan Choices

1. YOUR PERSONALIZED FOOD PLAN

The *Sweet Life Wellness* Personalized Food Plan is one of the easiest ways to lose weight because you make lower calorie substitutions by eating less of your usual foods and beverages. For example, a simple way to reduce your calories is to eat half as much as you do now at lunch or dinner. This kind of change doesn't require giving up any specific foods or necessarily mean changing the amount of fat, protein or carbohydrates you eat, and it's easy to remember.

You can make the personal food plan a heart healthy food pattern when you eat:

- ✧ Fewer foods that contain saturated fats
- ✧ More foods that are higher in fiber
- ✧ More fruit and vegetables
- ✧ Modify portions to lose weight

The *Sweet Life Wellness* Personalized Food Plan is one that fits your lifestyle and includes enough of the foods you like to keep you from feeling hungry.

The key to this plan is that this is not a restrictive diet. You are in the driver's seat. You can eat anything you want—the question is how much and how often you choose specific foods. Using an app, you can gauge how much you can eat and still lose weight. A helpful weight loss goal is to lose one to two pounds a week. Each person has her or his own unique metabolism. Bear in mind that some people lose weight more easily than others. Some people may only be able to lose half a pound a week. (I'm one of them.) Our varying metabolism makes it especially important to tune into and align with your body's pace of losing weight.

2. MEDITERRANEAN DIET

The Mediterranean dietary pattern (commonly known as the Mediterranean Diet) emphasizes traditional foods from countries that border the Mediterranean Sea, like Greece. In the past, this area enjoyed some of the lowest rates of chronic diseases and the highest life expectancy rates in the world. This diet plan naturally includes foods that are heart healthy and features olive oil as the principal source of fat. The diet also prescribes moderate amounts of low-fat cheese and yogurt, fish, poultry, and eggs, and limits red meat to a few times a month. The Mediterranean Diet is not low in calories, so you can begin to customize this plan to meet your goals.

See the sample Mediterranean Diet 1,200- and 1,600-calorie menus in the companion guidebook that showcases typical foods from Mediterranean-bordering countries. The 1,200-calorie menu is designed for women and the 1,600-calorie menu is designed for men, although your specific calorie range may vary up or down. The best thing to do is to experiment until you find a calorie range that allows you to consistently lose weight each week. The menu is one among a myriad of ways to make up a satisfying Mediterranean Diet menu.

The Mediterranean Diet is a good choice if you are interested in adopting a heart healthy eating plan and enjoy foods from the Mediterranean region.[44]

3. DASH EATING PLAN

The DASH Eating Plan (Dietary Approaches to Stop Hypertension) is designed for preventing or treating high blood pressure, a condition that affects one in three Americans, and more than 60 percent of U.S. adults aged sixty years and older. The DASH eating plan is a good choice for persons who are concerned about preventing or managing high blood pressure and are interested in a structured food plan that limits meat, sweets, and sodium.

As with the Mediterranean Diet, the DASH diet is not low in calories. The DASH Eating Plan can be used at a reduced level of calories for weight loss. Consult with your health care provider if you are using DASH or any other weight loss program and are currently taking medication for high blood pressure. Why? After weight loss, you may require less high blood pressure medication.

See the sample DASH diet 1,200- and 1,600-calorie-a-day menu in the companion guidebook. These menus exemplify how to make up a satisfying DASH diet menu.[45]

There isn't a dietary pattern or food plan like DASH that works for everyone. What is most important is to choose a plan that will help you make permanent lifestyle changes. The specific type of food plan you choose is less important than following a low-calorie diet of not less than 1,000 calories a day along with an eating pattern that is low in saturated fat, dietary cholesterol, and high in fiber, with plenty of fruits and vegetables to make it heart healthy. Your chances of success at losing excess weight will also increase by getting more physical activity along with individual coaching or group education.

The Mediterranean Diet and DASH also are the foundation of sustainable weight management from an environmental perspective because they are largely plant-based. Both plans recommend plenty of fruits, vegetables, and whole grains supplemented with small amounts of poultry, fish, meats, and low- or non-fat dairy products. You can manage your weight, be healthier, and reduce your food carbon footprint to help slow climate change by eating a largely plant-based diet that is low in calories.

The Mediterranean Diet and DASH may be more challenging for people who are used to eating large amounts of meat, sweets, and salty foods. If this sounds like you, consider choosing the *Sweet Life Wellness* Personal Food Plan, which gives you greater flexibility in making food choices that fit your current eating pattern.

Dietary Guidelines for Americans, 2020-2025

The Executive Summary of the latest *Dietary Guidelines for Americans* (DGA) astutely begins with, "The foods and beverages that people consume have a profound impact on their health."[46] The DGA aims to promote health and prevent disease by encouraging healthy eating patterns to:

- ✧ Meet nutrient needs
- ✧ Help achieve a healthy weight
- ✧ Reduce the risk of chronic disease

Why does the DGA emphasize achieving a healthy weight? In the US, currently nearly 75 percent of adults have weight issues either from being overweight or obese, which puts them at risk of developing chronic conditions, like diabetes, that are diet-related. The bottom line is that most of us eat too much highly processed food and don't get enough physical activity to avoid weight gain. But did you know that today, we have 600 more calories available per person in the United States each day than we did forty years ago? This means we are buying and eating larger portions of food, drinks, and calories than ever before. What we're eating and drinking, in many cases, is extremely out of kilter with what is recommended. For example, we eat foods with too much sugar, saturated fat, and sodium:

- ✧ 59% of US adult males and 63% of females eat more than the limit for the intake of added sugar

- ✧ 73% of adult males and 70% of females exceed recommendations for saturated fats

- ✧ 97% of adult males and 82% of females exceed the limit for sodium intake

Becoming Physically Active

Remember Janet and Steve, one of the couples I work with who each lost forty pounds this past year? They are partnering with me for a second year for support with weight maintenance. They go for a walk in the morning on most days. It never ceases to amaze them how much better they feel afterward. By the time they finish, they realize how much more alive they feel after a two- to three-mile walk. Among the long list of benefits of physical activity are being stronger and healthier, sleeping better, less likely to be depressed, and having a better chance of living longer.

Together, regular physical activity and making food choices selectively can help transport you to successfully meeting your weight management goals. Experts recommend increasing the amount you do gradually at first by increasing the amount of time you exercise and then the frequency. Did you know that physical activity can be a source of enjoyment and pleasure? Even a simple walk can become a highly enjoyable social or mentoring opportunity when you go with a friend or take your kids out for a hike or bike ride.

How Much Physical Activity Do You Need?

The current Physical Activity Guidelines for Americans recommend at least two hours and thirty minutes (150 minutes) each week of moderate aerobic physical activity (like brisk walking) to gain its many health benefits.[47] More is even better, and for weight management, persons who are most successful get an hour a day of aerobic physical activity.

These guidelines also include muscle-strengthening exercises for all muscle groups at least two days a week. According to the guidelines, the exercises for each muscle group should be repeated eight to twelve times per session.

How Can You Get Started?

It's easy to get started with physical activity when you are doing activities you enjoy and that fit your lifestyle. Some physical activity is better than none, and the more you do the better you feel. Many people begin with brisk walking.

The top five tips for getting started with physical activity are:

- ✧ Choose activities that you enjoy
- ✧ Find the times that work best for you
- ✧ If you are short on time, get physically active with whatever amount of time you can fit into your schedule and begin reaping health benefits
- ✧ Consider getting active with a buddy for inspiration and accountability
- ✧ Start at a comfortable pace

How Can You Uplevel Your Physical Activity?

Ready to do more? Build up gradually. First, add more time, and then increase frequency. Varying your workout will keep it fresh and fun. If you're already doing moderate physical activity like brisk walking, consider mixing it up by gradually adding in vigorous activities. Gradually increase the time you're active to five hours or more a week of moderate activity or the equivalent for even more health benefits.

HOW CAN YOU TELL THE DIFFERENCE BETWEEN MODERATE AND VIGOROUS LEVELS OF ACTIVITY?

Here are just a few moderate and vigorous aerobic physical activities:

Moderate Activities	Vigorous Activities
• Ballroom and line dancing	• Aerobic dance
• Biking on level ground or with few hills	• Biking faster than 10 miles per hour
• Canoeing	• Fast dancing
• General gardening (raking, trimming shrubs)	• Heavy gardening (digging, hoeing)
• Sports where you catch and throw (baseball, softball, volleyball)	• Hiking uphill
	• Jumping rope
• Tennis (doubles)	• Martial arts (such as karate)
• Using a manual wheelchair	• Race walking, jogging, or running
• Using hand cyclers— also called ergometers	• Sports with a lot of running (basketball, hockey, soccer)
• Walking briskly	• Swimming fast or swimming laps
• Water aerobics	• Tennis (singles)

Are you adding more time to your physical activity this week? If so, give yourself credit by recording your accomplishment on your ROADMAP Daily Action Plan.

Finding Your Own Pace to Lasting Weight Loss

Some people are on a fast track to weight loss while others prefer a gradual approach. What pace is right for you? What is needed is to align how quickly you want to lose weight with what you're willing to do to get there as well as your metabolism. More speed doesn't always yield greater success. Remember Aesop's Fable about the tortoise and the hare? The tortoise won the race by keeping a steady pace while the hare raced ahead and then fell behind when he stopped for a nap. A weight loss of one to two pounds a week is recommended by the National Institutes of Health.[48]

WARNING: very low-calorie diets of under 1,000 calories a day are not recommended because they require special monitoring and supplementation. The 1,200- and 1,600-calorie-a-day sample menus in this chapter were designed as a sample to guide you in creating a weight-loss food plan that can be adapted to fit different lifestyles, food tastes, and calorie levels. For example, if the calorie level on these menus doesn't seem right for you, adjust the menu up or down by a hundred calories a day and see if that works better for you.

WHAT IF YOU HAVE A LOT OF WEIGHT TO LOSE?

The *Sweet Life Wellness* Weight Loss Program is a comprehensive lifestyle approach that can be used if you have a significant amount of weight to lose. This program also can be combined with other weight loss methods. If you are obese (BMI of thirty or more) and believe you need a more aggressive approach, consider intensifying your efforts with dietary coaching with a registered dietitian, medications, and meal replacements. This program is not intended as a treatment for medical conditions, eating disorders, or psychological disorders. If you are obese and/or have one or more diet-related chronic health conditions, you may benefit from seeking the services of health care providers such as a registered dietitian, nurse practitioners, and physicians. A physician can provide medical monitoring. A registered dietitian can offer individual nutrition counseling and support to help you lose weight.

The principles and tools in the *Sweet Life Wellness* Weight Loss offer you the foundation for action and for building a healthy relationship with food and achieving long-term weight loss. Consider supplementing the tools offered in this program with support from your family, friends, colleagues, and buddies in the weight management program, and from health care providers. They can help build accountability, problem solving, and monitoring. Tell them that you are committed to losing weight and reaching your initial goal. Ask them to help support you in losing excess weight permanently.

Chapter Summary

This chapter is designed to help you build a healthy eating plan and physical activity plan that fit your lifestyle and desire for a happy life at a healthy weight. Three healthy eating plans are presented for you to select from. I also offer ideas about how to start or uplevel your physical activity, which can help you accelerate weight loss. I recommend that you go at your own pace with weight loss and adjust your approach if you have a lot of weight to lose.

Reflection Questions

1. Which of the three healthy eating plans introduced in this chapter will best fit your lifestyle?

2. What kind of physical activities do you enjoy?

3. When is the best time of day for you to be physically active?

How-To Guide

QUICK LIFE HACK

Looking at the Exercise: Sweet Life Wellness Personalized Food Plan Worksheet, what is one change you can easily make right now? Make that your next tiny change.

GUIDEBOOK EXERCISES

Exercise 21: *Sweet Life Wellness* Personalized Food Plan Worksheet
Resource 3: Sample One Day Menus—Mediterranean and DASH

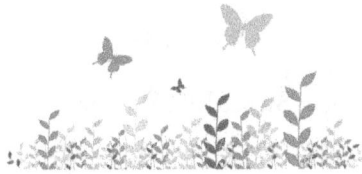

CHAPTER 21

Your Guide to Eating Out and Carry Out

WHEN DENISE FIRST CALLED ME, she told me that her weight had crept up and now it was affecting her health. She had pre-diabetes and diabetes ran in her family. She'd lost weight before and always gained it back. She didn't want to fall back into unhealthy habits, regain weight, and stop exercising after losing twenty pounds like she'd done before. One of the things she struggled with when eating out was making healthy food choices. Food was a big part of her social life, and she didn't want to feel that she couldn't enjoy food while eating out or going to parties. We did an assessment and found that she ate out several times a week: a couple lunches and once a week for dinner.

Denise began making changes and losing weight. Four months later, she said that what helped the most was that she wasn't eating out as much and was choosing vegetables more often at restaurants. When she went to parties, she was very selective about what she ate and what she decided to skip. When eating out at a restaurant, she cut her meal in half, asked for a box where she put half the meal before she even started eating so that it was out of sight. She found that she still enjoyed what she ate at restaurants as much as before and had the rest of the meal available to eat the next day.

Like Denise, maybe you want to have a strategy for making healthy choices while eating out. Why? Eating out poses a big challenge to weight loss success because portions are large and laden with sugar, salt, and fat and can undo much of the other good choices you make unless handled with care. Certain cuisines and types of restaurants offer more of these challenges than others. Fast food and casual dining restaurants, Chinese, Indian, Mexican, and barbeque restaurants can put a big dent in your intention to lose weight and keep it off. Let's first look at nutrition information available online or in restaurants. Then we'll offer you some ideas for creating your own Eating Out Game Plan.

Restaurant Nutrition Information

Did you know that some restaurant chains are required to disclose the number of calories for each item on their menus? This requirement applies to restaurant chains that have twenty or more locations doing business under the same name. The requirement can make deciding what to eat easier when dining out. Still, most restaurants are still loading on the calories, and "being choosy" can pay off when dining out. See below for some real surprises.

Calorie Sticker Shock

How can you avoid calorie "sticker shock" when eating out? Compare the items in the two lists below and you'll notice the wide variety of calories on chain restaurant menu items.

These ten items top the calorie heap:

Chili's Bacon Rancher Burger with Fries	2,200 calories
Baja Fresh Nachos with Steak	1,620
IHOP, Big Country Breakfast	1,280
Macaroni Grill, Parmesan Crusted Chicken	1,790
Applebee's Neighborhood Nachos with Chicken	1,830
Arby's Roast Turkey and Swiss Sandwich	1,645
Dairy Queen, six Chicken Strips with French Fries	1,580
Burger King Triple Whopper with Cheese	1,380
Macaroni Grill, Tiramisu	600
Baskin Robbins Chocolate Chip Cookie Dough Shake	1,140

These ten foods are lower calorie choices:

Applebee's 8 oz Steak with Garlic Mashed Potatoes	690 calories
Boston Market Chicken Caesar Salad with Dressing	770
Taco Bell Bean Burrito	350
Arby's Classic Roast Beef	360
Starbucks Ham and Swiss on a Baguette	480
Subway, Turkey Breast 6 inch Sub	280
Burger King Hamburger	260
Chick-fil-A Market Salad with Apple Vinaigrette	440
Baja Fresh Grilled Mahi Mahi Taco	230
Pizza Hut, 1/8 of 12 inch Veggie Lover's Pizza	200

Want to get the facts before going to a local restaurant? Consider viewing a restaurant's website for a rundown of their calories. Check for specific food items at large chain restaurant websites or at http://CalorieKing.com.

What's in a Name?

Did you notice that most of the menu items on the "top of the heap" calorie list above had more descriptive names? Think names like "parmesan crusted." Here's a story about the importance of naming menu items. Director of the Cornell University Food and Brand Lab Brian Wansink conducted a study at Bevier Cafeteria in Urbana, Illinois. He described the results of this study in his book, *Mindless Eating*.[49]

Researchers took six different foods in the cafeteria, and then offered each dish under two different names. They rotated foods on and off menus to avoid raising suspicion. For example, one day a menu item would be offered under the more mundane name of "Red Beans and Rice" and two weeks later the same dish was listed under the more descriptive name of "Traditional Cajun Red Beans and Rice."

What happened? The foods with more positive descriptions yielded 27 percent more sales. Diners also rated menu items with more interesting descriptors as "more appealing" and "tastier" than the identical foods with a boring name.

The results of this study can put us on "red alert" when we see food items with intriguing-sounding names. These are items that restaurants deem as more profitable, and they also may contain more calories.

Your Eating Out Game Plan

If you eat out often, having a game plan for eating out can help guarantee that you'll take action to meet your weight loss goals. How can you enjoy eating out without using up your day's calorie supply on just one meal? Try picking your top three strategies for dining out by creating Your Eating Out Game Plan below.

Chapter Summary

This chapter highlights the challenges posed to your weight loss success from eating out and carry out. I've shared some clues about what to watch out for when eating out about which meals may be better choices and given you a tool, the Your Eating Out Game Plan, to navigate this tricky terrain on your weight loss journey.

Reflection Questions

1. How often and where do you eat out or carry out from each week?

2. What is the impact of eating out and carry out on your ability to lose weight and keep it off?

3. What is one step you can take to manage your habit of frequently eating out and/or carry out that will help you accelerate your weight loss success (if this problem applies to you)?

How-To Guide

QUICK LIFE HACK

When eating out at a restaurant, ask for a box when you order and for it to be brought to the table when the food is served. Then, cut the meal in half, box up the second half, enjoy your meal, and take the box home, which gives you a meal for the next day.

GUIDEBOOK EXERCISES

Exercise 22: Your Eating Out Game Plan

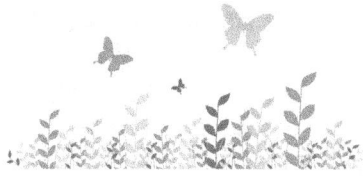

CHAPTER 22

Summary of Tough Weight Loss Challenges

THIS LIFESTYLE GUIDE IS DESIGNED to help you turn good intentions into action. Like Denise (who you met in Chapter 21) and Jeanette (in Chapter 14), many of my clients struggle with similar challenges. Denise struggled with making healthy menu choices when eating out. Jeanette suffered from being sleep-deprived from an overloaded work schedule. The remedy for both Denise and Jeanette was to make some decisions ahead of time and then implement them in their daily lives.

Challenges like eating out and getting enough sleep are addressed in this chapter. I highlight and help you pinpoint your toughest weight loss challenges and practical ways to solve them that you may not have implemented successfully yet. Some of these challenges were introduced in Part 1 as part of the ROADMAP Assessment Quiz. Please take this quiz to help you identify your top challenge. Several of the ideas in this section will amplify topics already covered in a *Happy Life at a Healthy Weight*.

Handling Tough Weight Management Challenges

Now, let's delve further into the toughest challenges that you've likely encountered on your way to building a healthy relationship with food and a healthy lifestyle.

1. Eating Out and Carry Out: Many restaurants pack a whole day's worth of calories (often more) into the meals they serve. Look at restaurant nutrition information online for some jaw dropping facts. For example, a serving of fish and chips at the Cheesecake Factory packs a whopping 1,860 calories. A piece of their original cheesecake is 830 calories. How can you eat out without sabotaging your weight loss? IDEA: Check online for restaurant menu and nutrition information before you choose a restaurant and use their online nutrition to choose what you'll eat before you go (or order out). See Chapter 21 for more about how to find delicious ways to enjoy eating out without sacrificing your weight loss goals by creating your own Eating Out Game Plan offered as a Guidebook Exercise at the end of this chapter. Mentally rehearsing your game plan before you leave for the restaurant can make for a delightful and guilt-free dining experience.

2. Food Shopping: Shopping with a list and going shopping when you're not hungry are tried and true tips for avoiding high-calorie splurges at the grocery store. What about buying foods in large containers at food warehouses? Brian Wansink concluded in his book *Mindless Eating* that, "You can certainly save money at the cash register, but you lose much of that money if you end up overbuying and having to throw food out .... Last, you can end up gaining weight by eating a food that you don't even like." This chapter offers you tips on becoming more selective about the foods and beverages you buy.

3. Planning for Special Occasions: Why think ahead about upcoming special occasions such as parties, celebrations, and vacations? With a little preparation, you'll be well equipped to avoid the pitfalls that can come with eating as part of a large group. Did you know that when seven or more people eat together, they tend to eat almost twice as much as they would if they were dining alone? Scope out ways ahead of time that you can successfully navigate situations when you're away from your usual routines. Then, five minutes before you leave, imagine yourself at the party (for example) and see yourself making choices that align with your weight loss intentions. Whatever the occasion, you can decide what foods to eat and which to skip to stay on track with your weight loss journey.

4. Getting a Good Night's Sleep: Getting enough sleep can help you follow through on your resolve to lose weight. Tired much of the time? Then, adapt the Tips for a Good Night's Sleep in Chapter 14 to your needs.

5. Relationships: Relationships can often support you in meeting your weight management goals. Still, there may be a person or two in your life who has good intentions but needs a direct request. Ask for what you need by saying, "Can I count on you to support my weight management program by (insert desired action)?"

6. Manage Emotions and Stress: In Chapter 14, I recommended ways to address chronic stress. However, there are also tumultuous times in life when emotions can become overwhelming due to illness or a family death. These times call for responding with flexibility and being forgiving with yourself. In such circumstances, decide what is best for you and your family, realizing that you can come back to your weight loss program when the crisis passes.

7. What to Do When Motivation Flags: Maybe you're bored with your eating or physical activity routine, and it's time to change it up. Maybe what you're doing doesn't match your lifestyle and you need to bring them into alignment. Take a look inside and see what you want and what you're willing to do to get there, and then adjust your expected results. Chapters 11 and 17 offer ways to instill motivation and inspire action.

8. Setbacks: Go easy on yourself when things don't go your way and you feel disappointed by setbacks. Prepare for such eventualities by writing a letter of encouragement to yourself (see the Guidebook Exercises at the end of this chapter) that will be ready for you to read when you're discouraged or feel like giving up on weight loss. What a generous gift you'll have given to yourself!

Food Shopping for Real Foods without Loading on the Calories

How can you navigate the miles and piles of foods when you shop without buying extras that lead to overeating? After all, according to the Food Marketing Institute, most supermarkets in 2022 carried nearly 32,000 items on average.[50] Have you thought about keeping it simple and buying authentic foods instead of industrial food products? Here are two tips:

1. Pick foods mostly from the periphery of the store where most of the "real" foods are located, like produce, meats, poultry, and dairy products.

2. Look at the ingredient labels and put "real" foods in your cart that have few ingredients. It can be just that simple.

Do you Know What's in the Foods You Buy?

Browsing ingredient lists is a shortcut to deciding whether the food is "real" or an industrial "food product."

Question: Which of these two examples is an "industrial food product?"

Example 1: Old Fashioned Oats

Ingredients: 100% Whole Grain Rolled Oats.

Example 2: Hidden Valley Ranch Dressing

Ingredients:

Vegetable oil (soybean and/or canola), water, buttermilk, sugar, salt, egg yolk, natural flavors, less than 1% of dried garlic, dried onion, vinegar, phosphoric acid, xanthan gum, modified food starch, monosodium glutamate, artificial flavors, disodium phosphate, sorbic acid and calcium disodium as EDTA as preservatives, disodium inosinate, and disodium guanylate.

Answer: The Hidden Valley Ranch Dressing is an "industrial food product" with a long list of chemical sounding ingredients.

Contrast the long list of ingredients in the commercial ranch dressing with a simple salad dressing made from extra virgin olive oil, ground pepper, and vinegar or lemon.

The Nutrition Facts Label: A Guide to Food Choices

What comes to mind when you think about making good food choices? How about food labels? In order to make good food choices, one needs to have an understanding of food labels. The aim is to help you gain a more in-depth understanding of the new nutrition facts label. The nutrition facts label can help with understanding how many calories and other nutrients are in a serving.

First things first: what information can you find on a nutrition facts label? According to the US Food and Drug Administration (FDA), some of the basic information (as shown in the pictures provided) includes: the serving information, the calories, the nutrients, and the percent daily value.[51] Some differences between the old and new labels, as stated by the FDA, include: the print of the servings and calories being larger and bolder, the addition of the added sugars section, and a new footnote.

As you go through a side-by-side comparison of reduced fat milk (2 percent low fat) and nonfat milk (sourced by USDA) with this new food label, I will provide a brief explanation of each of the four components, as well as how that information can be used to help make good food choices and help with weight loss.

In the example nutrition facts labels provided, you see:

✧   Nonfat milk has fewer calories, total fat, saturated fat, and cholesterol, than the reduced fat milk

✧   Nonfat milk has more Vitamin D and potassium than the reduced fat milk

With how the different components are labeled, it makes it easy to compare the macronutrients, micronutrients, serving sizes, etc., that are in the food item. This can be a benefit to those who are trying to be mindful of what they're eating.

Serving sizes are based on reference amounts commonly consumed by Americans.[52] As the FDA states, "it is not a recommendation of how much you should eat or drink." Just because a serving size is eight ounces doesn't mean that you *must* consume eight ounces. The rest of the label (i.e., amount of calories, macronutrients, micronutrients, percentage of daily value (%DV), etc.) is dependent on the serving size, so it is important to make sure that you pay attention to it. This is especially so as there's often more than one serving size in a container, but people may not pay attention to the serving size and believe the

REDUCED FAT MILK WITH ADDED VITAMINS A AND D	FAT FREE MILK WITH ADDED VITAMINS A AND D

Nutrition Facts

About 8 servings per container
Serving size 1 cup (240mL)

Amount per serving

Calories 130

	% Daily Value*
Total Fat 5g	6%
Saturated Fat 3g	15%
Trans Fat 0g	
Polyunsaturated Fat 0g	
Monounsaturated Fat 1.5g	
Cholesterol 20mg	7%
Sodium 135mg	6%
Total Carbohydrate 13g	5%
Dietary Fiber 0g	0%
Total Sugars 12g	
Includes 0g Added Sugars	0%
Protein 8g	16%

Vitamin D 2.5mcg 15% • Calcium 320mg 25%
Iron 0mg 0% • Potassium 420mg 8%
Vitamin A 150mcg 15% • Riboflavin 0.4mg 30%
Vitamin B12 1.3mcg 50% • Phosphorus 240mg 20%

*The % Daily Value (DV) tells you how much a nutrient in a serving of food contributes to a daily diet. 2,000 calories a day is used for general nutrition advice.

Nutrition Facts

About 8 servings per container
Serving size 1 cup (240mL)

Amount per serving

Calories 90

	% Daily Value*
Total Fat 0g	0%
Saturated Fat 0g	0%
Trans Fat 0g	
Polyunsaturated Fat 0g	
Monounsaturated Fat 0g	
Cholesterol <5mg	1%
Sodium 135mg	6%
Total Carbohydrate 13g	5%
Dietary Fiber 0g	0%
Total Sugars 12g	
Includes 0g Added Sugars	0%
Protein 8g	16%

Vitamin D 4.5mcg 25% • Calcium 300mg 25%
Iron 0mg 0% • Potassium 430mg 10%
Vitamin A 150mcg 15% • Riboflavin 0.4mg 30%
Vitamin B12 1.3mcg 50% • Phosphorus 250mg 20%

*The % Daily Value (DV) tells you how much a nutrient in a serving of food contributes to a daily diet. 2,000 calories a day is used for general nutrition advice.

INGREDIENTS: MILK, NONFAT FLUID, WITH ADDED VITAMIN A AND D	INGREDIENTS: MILK, NONFAT FLUID, WITH ADDED vitamin A AND D

information on the label refers to the container in its entirety. This can lead to the consumption of an excess amount of calories, protein, fat, carbs, sugars, and more.

Calories tell you how much energy you can obtain from eating a serving size of said food item. How many serving sizes you eat directly correlates to how many calories you consume. As each person's calorie needs differ, you want to make sure that you know your needs. For those who may be trying to lose weight, reading the nutrition label can prove beneficial as it helps you keep track of what you're eating. But keep in mind that calories aren't everything! You want to make sure that you are eating balanced and healthy meals. How you get your calories is just as important as how many calories you consume.

Percent Daily Value (%DV) is an important factor because it lets you know what percentage of your daily needs are met by a serving of this particular product. The FDA states that: "the %DV is the percentage of the daily value for each nutrient in a serving of the food. The daily values are reference amounts (expressed in grams, milligrams, or micrograms) of nutrients to consume or not to exceed each day. The %DV shows how much a nutrient in a serving of a food contributes to a total daily diet."

Take a look at the carbohydrates of the nonfat milk nutrient label, for example. According to the %DV, a serving size of that specific milk would provide 25 percent of the daily calcium requirement/limit based on a 2,000 calorie/day diet. It is important to know how to read and interpret this %DV as it can differ with brand and different conditions may require less or more consumption of certain nutrients (i.e. someone with heart disease or high blood pressure may be prescribed a low sodium diet).

Nutrients are an important part of the label because it's not just calories, fats, protein, and carbohydrates that you need to be aware of. This section of a nutrition facts label includes saturated fat, sodium, total sugars and added sugars, dietary fiber, vitamins, calcium, iron, and potassium.

Added sugars are those added during the processing stage, meaning they do not occur naturally in the food. To help prevent excessive or unwanted weight gain, it is important to look out for things like added sugars, sodium, saturated fat, etc. This is one of the benefits of nutrient labels—you can to pick and choose the foods that have more of the things you want and less of the things you don't according to your health goals and/or dietary needs

All in all, reading and understanding nutrition facts labels before buying, consuming, and/or preparing foods can help you to make better food choices. And with better choices, you can positively affect your health and move forward to reaching the goals you have planned.

Chapter Summary

This chapter highlights the toughest weight loss challenges I've encoun-tered for myself over decades and with my clients over the last twelve years of supporting adults with weight loss and nutrition related health problems. This chapter amplifies topics already covered in this book and offers practical ways to overcome those challenges that you may not yet have implemented successfully.

Reflection Questions

1. What new lifestyle changes have you made that are going well so far to help you lose weight?

2. Which lifestyle changes have you attempted that aren't going as well?

3. Which of these changes are the easiest and the hardest that you intend to commit to changing?

How-To Guide

QUICK LIFE HACK

If you get tired during the day, consider taking a twenty-minute power nap. This kind of nap refreshes, while a longer nap may leave you feeling groggy.

GUIDEBOOK EXERCISES

Exercise 23: My Toughest Weight Loss Challenge
Exercise 24: Letter of Encouragement

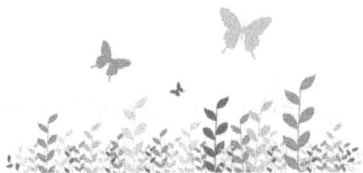

CHAPTER 23

Phases of Weight Loss and Weight Maintenance

WHERE ARE YOU ON YOUR WEIGHT LOSS JOURNEY and what's next for you? One thing for sure is that lasting weight loss success requires a long-term success strategy. Take Sophie as an example. Sophie needed to lose twenty pounds when she first called me. We assessed where to begin with making small changes. Her first habit changes were that she biked around her neighborhood with a friend every other evening and ate less for dinner during the week. She lost twenty pounds in twelve weeks. Sophie did well when she had the support of a buddy and participated in group weight loss sessions.

A few months after completing her weight loss program, Sophie's friend moved away, and she quit biking. She began to drink a glass of wine each evening. Gradually Sophie regained ten pounds of the weight she had lost. Sophie felt disappointed, yet she learned something from her relapse. Temporary dieting wasn't the answer. She needed a plan and continued support to stick with a program that would help her with both weight loss and maintenance. She returned to the Sweet Life Wellness Weight Loss Program and this time lost a total of twenty pounds and kept it off. Sophie's story is an example of why people who want to lose weight need a plan for both the weight loss and weight maintenance phases of weight loss.

Growth Mindset for Weight Loss Success

In Chapter 8, I shared Carol Dweck's approach to mindset with you. A Stanford University psychologist, Dweck discovered and researched a groundbreaking idea that led to her book, *Mindset, The New Psychology of Success*. Rather than one global mindset, as Dweck explained, our mindset differs depending on the activity. Dweck explained two different types of mindsets that people carry about specific issues. The first is a fixed mindset, one that assumes that intelligence is static and either you have it or you don't. The other possibility is a growth mindset, one that comes with a belief that intelligence can be developed. As mentioned in Chapter 8, people with a fixed mindset believe that losing weight means being strong and using willpower. On the other hand, people with a growth mindset know that they can learn and apply new strategies to lose weight and keep it off.

Why is mindset important while losing weight and even more important when keeping it off? With a fixed mindset, people tend to make an earnest and superficial effort at weight loss and then hope for the best. Then, they beat themselves up when they fail. Persons with a growth mindset make a special effort and apply effective strategies and systems to make change happen.

The difference in the two mindsets can make all the difference in whether a person is able to lose and maintain weight loss. Persons with a growth mindset are more likely to continue the strategies that made them successful with weight loss in the first place. **Unfortunately, many people stop the behaviors that made them successful with weight loss after they have lost the weight.** Vulnerabilities continue, and you'll need to continue using the same success strategies you used for losing weight if you expect lasting results.

Phases of Weight Loss and Weight Maintenance

Let's briefly look at the five phases of weight loss and weight maintenance and what each phase means. We will also pinpoint when it's time to move from one phase to another.

PHASE 1: WEIGHT GAIN

Increased weight gain over the last several decades has caused almost three-quarters of Americans to become overweight or obese. The reason this weight gain is important is because overweight and obesity lead to increased risk of diabetes and other conditions, decreased mobility, and the inability to be able to do the things you want to do in life. Each year millions of individuals attempt to lose weight, and most of them don't succeed in the long run. If this sounds like you, you're looking for a way to lose weight *and* keep it off.

PHASE 2: INITIAL WEIGHT LOSS

Success at weight loss begins with changing habits. Changing habits starts with knowing why you want to lose weight and who you want to be. Then, weight loss results from applying new habits that you can sustain. Beginning steps might include deciding to:

- Identify who you want to become and how living a happy life at a healthy weight will support your vision
- Discover and tap into your top reasons for losing weight
- Choose an initial and long-term weight goal
- Renew yourself to release stress and build resilience
- Create a viable food and physical activity plan
- Monitor your food and drink intake

If you haven't already done so, take the ROADMAP Assessment Quiz in Chapter 3. Then, choose how to navigate this book and address your most pressing inner roadblocks to living a happy life at a healthy weight. Remember that the initial weight loss phase will vary with the amount you want to lose.

PHASE 3: WEIGHT PLATEAU

A weight plateau phase may follow an initial weight loss of 5 to 10 percent of body weight. This is a phase where your body weight stabilizes and stays within the same two pounds, sometimes for an extended period. This phase often continues until you adopt new habits that disrupt a weight plateau. These are changes you can make, like adding more physical activity (type, time, and/or intensity) and other activities that promote a relaxation response, getting a good night's sleep, and changing the amount, type, or frequency of what you eat. A weight plateau may help your body adjust to a new weight and then signal that it is time to take on new habit changes.

PHASE 4: RENEWED WEIGHT LOSS

After losing and then reaching a weight plateau, you might decide on a new weight loss goal and what habit changes will help you get there.

PHASE 5: WEIGHT MAINTENANCE

The weight maintenance phase assumes success at reaching a weight you feel is right for you. This phase can be particularly tricky. Deliberate strategies are needed to successfully maintain the initial weight loss. Time is needed to consolidate and sustain your initial weight loss. See below for weight maintenance strategies.

Decision Points

When is the right time to transition from one weight loss phase to another?

1. Weight gain to weight loss: You've decided to change your lifestyle to lose weight and keep it off. You make enough small lifestyle changes that allow you to go beyond weight gain and weight plateau to losing weight.

2. Weight loss to weight maintenance: You are ready for a transition to weight maintenance because you've reached a weight that you are satisfied with and want to keep it off.

3. Weight plateau to weight maintenance: It's timely to transition from a weight plateau (a temporary phase) to weight maintenance (a permanent phase) when you've made all the changes you're willing to make, and you have reached a weight that is acceptable to you.

4. Weight maintenance to renewed weight loss: Are you ready to make more changes to lose weight? You'll know when the timing is right to add new habit changes. Then, you decide which lifestyle changes to make so you can step into renewed weight loss.

Weight Maintenance Strategies

The National Weight Control Registry currently tracks 10,000 people who have lost a significant amount of weight and have kept it off. Participants enrolled in this registry have lost at least thirty pounds and have kept it off for at least one year. How did participants maintain their weight? Participants reported that they lost and maintained their weight by making changes in their food intake and physical activity. Most continue to maintain a low-calorie, low-fat diet and a high level of physical activity. The most frequent activities that many of them continue are that they:

✧ Exercise on average an hour a day (90 percent)

✧ Eat breakfast every day (78 percent)

✧ Weigh themselves at least once a week (75 percent)

✧ Watch less than ten hours of television a week (62 percent)

What else is important to remember about successfully maintaining weight loss? Only a modest increase in calories is needed when switching from a weight loss phase to a weight maintenance phase.[53]

With the *Sweet Life Wellness* Weight Loss Program, I offer clients a twelve-month program that can be renewed, because it takes time to master habit change, lose weight, and keep it off. Some of us go for decades bouncing between weight loss and weight gain, usually by temporarily dieting. Eventually, we become disappointed if not downright discouraged. Instead, I offer you a comprehensive lifestyle change approach to weight loss that is focused on choosing habits to change and continually committing to them so they stick with you long-term.

Summary

The lifestyle changes covered in this guidebook are designed for you to adopt and commit to so that they become a permanent part of your lifestyle. These are tiny changes that can make a big difference over time. These changes are designed for your lasting success so you can live a happy life at a healthy weight. This kind of change requires renewing your commitment to apply new daily habits instead of letting complacency creep in that leads to relapse, weight plateau, and weight regain. This chapter describes the phases of weight loss and weight maintenance to help you cultivate the continued mindset and awareness that is needed to sustain positive results. In terms of mindset, this requires change from a *judge-and-be-judged* framework to a *learn-and-help-learn* framework. A change in mindset takes time, effort, and support. Using a growth mindset, you'll notice that you can discover new ways to grow and learn each day.

Reflection Questions

1. What phase are you in currently with your weight?

2. What are your choices and what will you do when you reach a weight plateau?

3. What mindset and strategies will help you transition to a weight maintenance phase?

How-To Guide

QUICK LIFE HACK

When transitioning from a weight loss phase to weight maintenance, increase your intake by 100-200 calories and experiment to see whether you still maintain weight with this change. If you are already at a weight plateau, you're already taking in the calories you need for weight maintenance. No increase in calories is needed.

GUIDEBOOK EXERCISES

Exercise 25: Creating a Plan for a Happy Life at a Healthy Weight

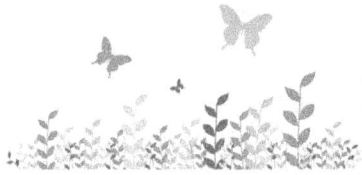

CHAPTER 24

Body Image, Healthy at Any Weight

This chapter co-authored with Emma O'Connor

SOME CLIENTS FOCUS ON THEIR DESIRE to stop being controlled by food, behavior change, and healthy eating rather than on weight loss. Take Shelly, for example. After she called and we did a follow-up assessment, she told me about a painful experience she had in childhood with her weight. Her mother had an eating disorder and often made her daughter get on the scale and then shamed Shelly about her weight. This meant that when Shelly called me, she said that she didn't want the number on the scale to be a primary indicator of success and she did want help with emotional eating. She was willing to track her weight and declared that she wanted to look at things like consistency, mood, and energy instead of weight as the main success factors. This approach worked well for Shelly. She lost twenty-five pounds as a result of the positive lifestyle changes she made, with her primary result being her increased self-compassion and satisfaction with her progress.

When Elle called me for help, she told me that she had lost weight before and had felt good but hadn't sustained the weight loss. When we did an assessment, she revealed that she felt that the prevalent paradigm of shaming, especially of women to lose weight and eat healthy, contributed to her feeling trapped by shame. Now in her fifties, she wanted to find a new path to healthy eating and activity so she could be healthy physically and mentally and feel comfortable in her body again at whatever size that might be. She wanted to be out of the trap of the prevailing shame paradigm and use the "health at every weight" viewpoint as a guide. As she started on a new path, she envisioned enjoying food without emotional eating. Then she changed her eating behaviors and increased her physical activity and created new healthier habits. Six months later, she began tracking and gradually losing weight after she felt comfortable adding this dimension to her lifestyle change approach.

The central theme of this book is to inspire you to take a stand and empower yourself to live the life you want with well-being, compassion, and self-care. It is designed to help you build a healthy relationship with food and a healthy lifestyle to get there. Discovering who you want to become, coupled with a lifestyle change process to help you get there, guides your journey to a desired destination of being happy at any weight. By design, we recommend that you are primarily concerned with your happiness, well-being, and habit change with a secondary focus on weight—your happy life is the central focus and a healthy weight comes along with it.

In a world that often prioritizes a certain body image as the epitome of beauty, it's crucial to challenge these standards and embrace being healthy at any weight. This chapter delves into the significance of body positivity, dispelling myths surrounding weight and health, and highlighting the importance of self-love and acceptance. Developing healthy and sustainable habits can contribute to physical and mental well-being and a healthier lifestyle, leading to a more sustainable and fulfilling approach to achieving personal weight goals.

Body positivity is a movement that advocates for the acceptance and celebration of all body types, regardless of societal norms or standards. It promotes the idea that every individual deserves to feel comfortable and confident in their own skin, no matter what their size, shape, or weight may be at the time.

One common misconception is that a lower weight automatically equates to better health. However, this oversimplification neglects the complexity of health, which involves various factors such as genetics, lifestyle, and mental well-being. Exploring the importance of forming healthy habits with food before diving right into weight loss can provide a sustainable lifestyle that will eventually lead to weight goals.

A holistic approach to health considers mental well-being alongside physical health. Constantly striving for an unrealistic body ideal can lead to stress, anxiety, and other mental health issues. Embracing one's body at any weight contributes to improved mental well-being and fostering a positive relationship with oneself.

Practicing these tips can help foster this empowering perspective:

Practice Self-Love and Acceptance

✧ Celebrate your body for its uniqueness and the incredible things it allows you to do

✧ Focus on positive affirmations and challenge negative thoughts about your body

Shift the Focus to Healthful Behaviors

✧ Concentrate on adopting healthy habits, then if and when it makes sense for you, create a target weight goal that motivates and inspires you

✧ Prioritize nourishing your body with a balanced and varied diet

Practice Mindful Eating

✧ Pay attention to hunger and fullness cues and eat with intention and awareness

✧ Savor and enjoy your meals without judgment, promoting a positive relationship with food

Engage in Regular Physical Activity

✧ Find enjoyable forms of exercise that make you feel good, whether it's walking, dancing, or yoga

✧ Shift the focus from exercise as a means of weight loss to an activity that enhances your well-being, such as improved flexibility, increased energy, or better sleep

✧ Celebrate small victories and progress towards a healthier lifestyle

Educate Yourself

✧ Stay informed about the complexity of health and the limitations of using weight as the sole indicator

✧ Explore resources that challenge societal norms and promote a more inclusive definition of health

Be Patient and Kind to Yourself

✧ Understand that change takes time, and fostering a positive body image is a journey

✧ Practice self-compassion and treat yourself with the same kindness you would offer to a friend

Your ROADMAP for Success is the foundational tool to guide your steps along the way to help you recognize that no matter what has happened to you, you have a choice to have a healthier lifestyle and stop being controlled by food. Start with healing the past by recognizing, forgiving, and releasing your root cause of shame that has become connected with food. We use this process to help you let go of shame and being controlled by food in the moment when you are triggered to eat. This journey is designed as a catalyst to your future abundance, joy, and health.

The intended result is to help you move from a place of shame and lower self-esteem to thriving. As a daily practice, this healing includes helping you stop using food as relief by listening to and accepting your feelings and embracing what you truly want instead of turning to food as consolation. How does it work? Nurturing yourself with a healthy diet, physical activity, and lifestyle behaviors and committing to these actions daily.

Chapter Summary

One misconception is the belief that a lower weight inherently equates to better health. This perspective neglects the complexity of health, considering factors such as genetics, lifestyle, and mental well-being. This chapter emphasizes the importance of a holistic approach to health, incorporating mental well-being alongside physical health. Constantly striving for an unrealistic body ideal can lead to stress, anxiety, and other mental health issues. Embracing one's body at any weight improves mental well-being, fostering a positive relationship with oneself.

Reflection Questions

1. How has societal pressure influenced your perception of body image, and how can you challenge these influences?

2. In what ways do you prioritize your mental well-being alongside your physical health?

3. How can you shift your focus from pursuing a specific weight goal to adopting healthier habits?

4. Reflect on your small victories and progress towards a healthier lifestyle. How do these achievements contribute to your overall well-being?

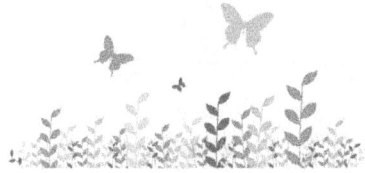

CHAPTER 25

Environmentally Sound Lifestyle Choices

"Widespread and rapid changes in the atmosphere, ocean, cryosphere, and biosphere have occurred. Human-caused climate change is already affecting many weather and climate extremes in every region across the globe. This has led to widespread adverse impacts and related losses and damages to nature and people." IPCC Report 2023[54]

JOANIE WAS ON A KETO DIET when she called me for help with weight loss. She kept her carbohydrates to a minimum by eating vegetables like cauliflower, kale, and celery, as well as snack foods and desserts like tortilla chips, ice cream sundaes, and candy. Her diet was high in protein and fat, especially saturated fats. Most of the fat and protein she ate came from animal-based foods like sausage, steak, pizza, chicken wings, butter, cheese, eggs, and bacon. She had previous success with this diet and was confident it would work again to help her lose weight and keep it off. As a client, she was unwilling to transition from the Keto diet to a flexible lifestyle weight-loss plan. During the first six months of her program, she lost twenty-five pounds. Eventually, she was unable to sustain the Keto diet and began regaining weight.

Then, her doctor commented that her blood lipid values had become too high. She learned that she was at risk for heart disease. Unfortunately, the extremely popular Keto diet is both hard to sustain and comes with serious risks. Only short-term results have been studied and nothing is known for sure about whether it's safe in the long term. What is the Keto diet? Keto is one of several weight loss diets that are low in carbohydrates and high in protein, along with the Paleo, Atkins, and South Beach diets. What makes Keto different is that most calories come from fat and protein. Carbohydrates are restricted to 5 percent of calories.

The other dimension Joanie hadn't considered was the impact of the animal products she was eating and their contribution to greenhouse gas (GHG) emissions and climate change. Joanie's example brings up three problems with the Keto (and other low carbohydrate) diets. The problems with these diets are that:

1. They are high in animal products and aren't usually sustainable in the long run for weight loss.
2. They can increase risk for health conditions like heart disease.
3. These diets also contribute to greenhouse gas emissions and climate change.

Food and Climate Change

The types and amounts of food we eat contribute to climate change through greenhouse gas emissions. Luckily, many changes we can make to eat healthier and manage our weight will help slow climate change. When we act together, we can create a tipping point. We have within our grasp the collective power to use sustainable practices that will help manage our weight and protect the Earth at the same time.

I created the signature *Sweet Life Wellness* weight loss program to offer environmentally friendly and health-enhancing weight loss options for people who are frustrated with short-term dieting and temporary results, want to build a healthy relationship with food, and who care about the planet.

What Is the Impact of Food on the Environment?

While we often hear environmentalists urge consumers to buy fuel-efficient cars or change to fluorescent or LED light bulbs to help protect the environment, we hear less about changing what kind and how much food we should eat. How and to what extent does our food system contribute to climate change? Based on this analysis, the food system is one of our planet's major users of carbon-rich sources of energy.

It's estimated that a third of all human-caused greenhouse gas emissions are linked to food. This number came from an assessment of global system GHG emissions that included food production, consumption, processing, transport, and packaging from the EDGAR-Food database, which estimated GHG emissions for 1990-2015.[55] Their estimate showed that food system emissions in 2015 accounted for 34 percent of total GHG emissions globally, with agriculture and land use activities like raising crops and animals making the largest contribution and supply chain activities, like transporting food, accounting for much of the rest.

While most discussions of food and the environment focus on changing the kinds of foods we eat, there is evidence that overeating and obesity also may contribute to greenhouse gas emissions that harm the environment. Researchers Phil Edwards and Ian Roberts at the London School of Hygiene and Tropical Medicine conducted an analysis and calculated that a country with 40 percent of the population who are obese would require 19 percent more energy from food production and transportation compared with a normal population distribution of body mass index (BMI).[56] This increase would result in greater greenhouse gas emissions. These findings suggest that reducing the amount of food you eat as you lose weight and keep it off is also good for the planet.

How Can I Help Reduce GHG Emissions with Lifestyle Choices?

The foods that have the greatest impact on GHG emissions come largely from agriculture and land use activities described above.[57] With this in mind, you can make a few straightforward dietary choices that will have a big impact on your personal carbon footprint, such as:

- ✧ Eating more plant-rich meals and fewer meals with animal-based products like meat and diary

- ✧ Planning your meals so that you reduce the amount of food you throw out

- ✧ Trying recipes made with local and seasonal foods

- ✧ Avoiding plastic packaging and single-use plastic bags in your shopping and food storage

Another simple step you can take to help reduce climate change is to shop for foods that have a simple list of ingredients, because they require less processing and energy use in their production. Many of these steps are a part of everyday consumer choices. Gidon Eshel and Pamela Martin of the Department of Geophysical Sciences, University of Chicago noted in an article on diet and climate change that by switching from red meat to poultry or eggs or plant-based foods, you can help with reducing your carbon footprint by as much as driving a hybrid instead of a solely gas-fueled car."[58]

How Can I Eat Green, Lose Weight, and Keep It Off?

In reviewing the connection between food and climate change, I discovered that three factors that promise to help reduce GHG emissions are vital to successful long-term weight management.

These factors are:

✧ How much we eat

✧ The types of foods we select

✧ The ways we prepare and store food

Five Tips for Eating Green and Losing Weight

My top five tips for eating green *and* losing weight, based primarily on my review of the research related to food system contributions to greenhouse gas emissions, are:

1. Shift to eating a more plant-based diet with smaller amounts of animal foods, especially red meat and dairy. For protein options: eat red meat less often and reduce portions to three to four ounces a serving. Replace these proteins where possible with legumes (beans), tofu, chicken, and eggs, which are more energy efficient. Eat meatless and dairy-free meals for dinner at least once a week.
2. Buy and eat more fruit and vegetables.
3. Eat more whole grains.
4. Reduce food waste.
5. Adjust food portion sizes and reduce your calories from food and beverages to help you lose weight and keep it off.

Food, Lifestyle, and Weight Gain Over the Decades

Food has become more affordable over the decades. The United States produces more food than ever, making it easy to see why so many of us have gained weight. Even with food becoming relatively less expensive, Americans have shown a strong preference for low-cost refined grains, fats, and sweets that are high in calories. We eat vast amounts of highly processed industrial food products like chips and soft drinks that cost less and are convenient yet offer little more than fat, sugar, salt, and chemical ingredients.

The fascinating story of David Wallerstein illustrates how the food industry learned that we eat more when they give us more. He experimented with ways to boost popcorn sales in movie theaters in the Midwest and discovered that when he introduced jumbo sizes, popcorn sales skyrocketed.[59] McDonald's Corporation founder Ray Kroc adopted Wallerstein's idea and discovered the lucrative business strategy of supersizing. As a result, many foods became super-sized. Today's soda is nearly triple the size and number of calories as a soda of twenty years ago. Today's plain bagel serves up twice as many calories. No wonder Americans have gotten heavier and heavier, and climate change has accelerated.

We continue to eat more highly processed foods and our average daily calorie intake continues to climb. A USDA report showed that the total food available increased by 16 percent between 1970 and 2003.[60] This increase in the available food supply resulted in a jump in calories from 2,234 to 2,757 (after adjusting for plate waste, spoilage, and other food losses). Globally, calorie intake per person continues to climb, with the United States and Europe leading the way. Calorie intake per person in the US continues to increase and is now at 3,150 calories a day according to a UN News Report published in 2022.[61]

It's no secret that people take in more calories when eating out. More than half (55 percent) of Americans ate at restaurants on any given day as of 2018.[62] Restaurants make menu items irresistible by hyper-loading them with sugar, fat, and salt (think cheese fries and buffalo wings), as revealed in David Kessler's book, *The End of Overeating*.[63] According to Kessler, the food industry produces foods designed to hyper-stimulate our palate that have created a culture of overeating.

Highly processed food products purchased from grocery stores and restaurants (including dine-in and carry-out) have created an unhealthy food environment. Such foods contrast with the rich colors, tastes, and textures of real foods and meals prepared from a short list of simple, natural ingredients.

Still, what we eat is only a part of the story of continuing weight gain in the US. We are a nation of individuals who are largely inactive both at work and play. Why? Shifts in our economy from agriculture to the current information age have led to a dramatic decline in our need for individual physical energy expenditure. Ours is a life of physical conveniences, where most of us spend our waking hours sitting rather than moving. It comes as no surprise that we have intentionally engineered the need for most physical activity out of our lives. As a quick example, we take for granted that cars come with windows that roll up and down at the touch of a button. Who even remembers when windows were manually rolled up?

During annual visits to Europe in the last twenty years, I noticed how much more physically active people were as they went about their lives and how many fewer people were overweight or obese than in the United States. While vacationing in Paris and the Loire Valley, I marveled at women skipping along with their children along the Seine River in Paris and women in their fifties and sixties delivering mail on bicycle in Mont Louis Sur Loire, a suburb of Tours one hundred miles south of Paris. Almost a decade earlier, I had witnessed with envy the practice of the people who lived in Siena, Italy. Every evening, they took an evening stroll and greeted their neighbors.

Surprisingly, nearly three in four American adults are overweight or obese[64] and nearly half of them try to lose weight each year.[65] We are beginning to understand the consequences of obesity, from consumption of highly processed food products, inactivity, and less sleep. The epidemic of overweight and obesity in the United States exacts a high price on our health and in health care spending. For example, medical spending costs $1,861 more a year for an obese person than for persons of normal weight.[66] Treatment for diabetes and heart disease are among forty obesity-related medical conditions. These conditions contribute to medical costs for obesity that have nearly doubled in the last decade. Our collective food preferences for animal-based foods also contribute significantly to GHG emissions and climate change.

The sad fact is that we now have a new generation of overweight and obese children and adults who have increasing rates of chronic diseases like diabetes. The result of these increasing rates of chronic disease has reduced life expectancy in the US. We can do better. Alarmingly, the United States ranks first in the percentage of people who are overweight and obese among industrialized Organization for Economic Co-operation and Development (OECD) countries. Sadly, the United States ranks fourteenth among 223 countries worldwide for life expectancy.[67]

The damaging consequences of overweight and obesity and preferences for animal-based foods make it all the more compelling that we adopt sound practices for sustainable weight management based on the best available scientific evidence. On an optimistic note, we have an unprecedented opportunity and the time to act is now. The stakes are too high to justify using temporary diets and quick fixes when sound weight management and wellness practices are now available.

Chapter Summary

Five of the most important steps to lose weight and keep it off turn out to be the same steps that will significantly reduce climate change from greenhouse gas emissions. These steps are to:

- ✦ Eat a plant-based diet or reduce the amount of animal-based foods you eat. Eat smaller portions of meat, choose leaner varieties, and choose poultry and fish or eggs more often.

- ✦ Increase the amount of fruits, vegetables, and whole grains you eat. Generally, these foods are naturally low in calories and high in nutrients.

- ✦ As part of a low-calorie diet, pay attention to portion sizes and reduce the total amount of food you eat.

- ✦ Bring your own reusable bag while shopping and buy unprocessed foods that will help you lose weight while reducing food waste.

- ✦ Use your car less and burn calories with physical activity. For example, walk or bike on errands or food shopping in neighborhoods that are walkable.

Our collective choices make a significant difference because we live at a pivotal time in terms of climate change and in a highly connected world. Until now, we have used technology to exploit our resources and feed consumer demand for products. We have pushed the limits of locality and seasonality to such an extent that we have foods from all parts of the world at all times of the year. We are realizing the consequences of what we have gained in terms of climate change. Now is an unparalleled opportunity to collectively heal our relationship with food and the planet by making the relatively simple changes outlined in this chapter. These are choices that stand to benefit both our waistlines and the planet for the long term.

Reflection Questions:

1. Reflect on your dietary habits. How closely do they align with the recommendations for environmentally sound and healthy eating presented in the chapter?

2. Consider the information about food production, transportation, and waste. How might you adjust your shopping habits to contribute to reduced greenhouse gas emissions and lower your carbon footprint?

3. Evaluate your daily physical activity levels. How can you incorporate more movement into your routine, especially when running errands?

4. Explore the connections made between climate change and weight management. How does the chapter suggest that adopting sustainable practices for weight management can contribute to addressing climate change?

Reflect on the international perspective provided, particularly regarding the comparison of lifestyle and weight issues in the United States and Europe. How might cultural and societal factors influence lifestyle choices related to food and physical activity in different regions?

How to Guide

QUICK LIFE HACK

What is one easy change you could make to eat a more plant-based diet?

GUIDEBOOK EXERCISE

Exercise 26: Tips for Eating Green and Losing Weight

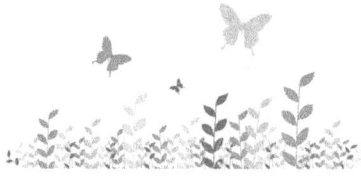

Conclusion

AFTER READING THIS BOOK, you've likely discovered that you no longer have to put up with diets that result in your weight going up and down time after time. Continuous weight cycling can be prevented. I've shown you how in this book. Instead, I believe that you deserve to live in the sweet spot of your life with a healthy mind and body at the weight you want to be. You deserve to live the life you've always wanted to live at the weight you want to be and look in the mirror and love who you see.

Who This Book Is For

This book is dedicated to you, adults who want to successfully lose weight and keep it off for a happy life at a healthy weight. You've likely tried dieting to lose weight, probably repeatedly. You're probably disappointed with the results and yourself. You're fed up with dieting. You yearn for a healthy relationship with food. You feel ashamed that you lose control, slide back to overeating, and have failed to find the right solution.

MAIN THEMES

With this book, I took you on a journey designed to be a catalyst for your future abundance, joy, and health. My aim is that with this journey you begin to build a healthy relationship with food so you can live the life you've always wanted to live at a healthy weight. My mission is to help you break free from food triggers and lifestyle choices that cause overeating. In doing so, this book emphasized healing the connection between food and shame. I am confident that you can free yourself from being controlled by food and overeating by continuing this journey. The intended result is to help you move from a place of shame about your relationship with food and your weight to thriving. This healing, as a daily practice, is designed as a way for you to stop using food as relief from stress and mood by listening to and accepting your feelings and embracing what you truly want instead of turning to food as consolation.

This book uses a problem-focused approach designed for you to avoid the trap that comes when you expect quick weight loss results and fall for a gimmicky short-term diet. Instead, I recommended empowering yourself to apply tiny behavior changes that can add up and make a big difference with a comprehensive lifestyle change approach.

As you've read this book, you probably noticed that I've encouraged you to become an advocate and take a stand for yourself. With this book, I've asked you to make your own rules. By now, I expect that you've defined what a healthy weight means for you. You have the tools in hand and may have begun to use the comprehensive lifestyle approach to habit change and weight loss outlined in this book. I recommend that you continue focusing on behavior changes that fit your lifestyle and that you can sustain. Most importantly, I have guided you through the weight loss and weight maintenance phases, because losing weight is easier than keeping it off. You have the tools in hand so you can continue to remove inner roadblocks and nurture yourself with conscious food choices, physical activity, and healthier lifestyle behaviors.

The behavior change approach used in this book is also relevant to other weight loss approaches, like surgery and medications. In fact, consistently making the better lifestyle choices outlined in this book are essential to to success, either with weight loss surgery or medications.

The Road Ahead

This book took you on a journey designed to help you discover and remove the inner and outer obstacles at play that prevent you from living a happy life at a healthy weight. I began by introducing you to the connection between food and shame in Part 1. The book highlighted the roots of shame and showed you how the cycle of overeating plays out in real life. By now you have taken the ROADMAP Assessment Quiz and found the starting point for your journey and a Success ROADMAP that equipped you to navigate your most important inner obstacles.

Part 2 was designed to help you remove the inner obstacles getting in your way. Each chapter offered a How-To Guide with practical tools to easily apply to your everyday life. A key tool I made available is the Five Steps to Stop Being Controlled by Food. I have successfully used this tool with many weight loss clients. Part 3, Lifestyle Guide to a Happy Life at a Healthy Weight, featured key practical ideas to put preferred solutions into practice in a way that fits your lifestyle.

Take Aways

You are on a continuing journey to live a happy life at a healthy weight. This book offers practical tools that you can easily apply to break free from food triggers and heal the connection between food and shame. The intended outcome of making recommended habit changes is to overcome inner and outer obstacles, lose weight, and keep it off. I wish you every success on your journey.

How to Get Your Companion Guidebook

A companion guidebook with more practical tools for applying the ideas and concepts in each chapter of this book is available. To receive access to your companion guidebook, visit https://www.sweetlifewellness.com/guidebook/.

What's Next

Coming soon! The online training program for Building a Healthy Relationship with Food will be available in 2024. When you request the companion guidebook, you'll also receive future notices about the availability of the online program.

How to get more help

To read the Sweet Life Wellness blog posts and watch videos by Kay Loughrey for additional tips, you can:

Visit the Sweet Life Wellness Website at: www.sweetlifewellness.com

Sign up for Kay Loughrey's YouTube Channel at: https://www.youtube.com/@kayloughrey6726

Client Stories by chapter

Julie	Introduction
Katie	Chapters 1 and 7
Janet and Steve	Chapters 5 and 16
Jenny	Chapter 6
Josie	Chapters 6 and 9
Jeanette	Chapters 8, 11, 14, and 22
Joanne	Chapter 9
Phil	Chapter 10
Michelle	Chapters 11 and 12
Max	Chapter 13
Laurel	Chapter 15
Justin	Chapters 16, 18, and 20
Doris	Chapter 17
Jennifer	Chapter 18
Leora	Chapter 18
Brent	Chapter 18
Sandy	Chapter 18
Joy	Chapter 19
Brandon	Chapter 19
Denise	Chapters 21 and 22
Sophie	Chapter 23
Shelly	Chapter 24
Elle	Chapter 24
Joanie	Chapter 25

Acknowledgements

WRITING THIS BOOK HAS BEEN A JOURNEY of discovery, growth, and profound gratitude. I would like to extend my heartfelt thanks to my village—the many people who have supported and contributed to this book's creation.

First and foremost, my deepest appreciation goes to my "First Readers"—Lori Pujols, Kimberly Cox, and Meghan Lucas. Your time, attention to detail, and invaluable insights have been instrumental in shaping this book. Meghan, your feedback and encouragement have made it richer and more impactful than I could have ever imagined.

I owe a huge debt of gratitude to Jo Schonewolf, my amazing right hand for the past year. Jo, your tireless work in taking the concepts and content of this book, and editing, formatting, and transforming them into other mediums has been extraordinary. Your dedication has made it possible to reach and help more people on a bigger scale and in more accessible ways. I hope you are present to your ripple effect.

To my incredible clients, thank you for your unwavering commitment to doing the hard work of uncovering the deep connections between past events, including big and small traumas, and weight loss issues - and being willing to bring me along for the ride! Your courage and perseverance are truly inspiring and have been a constant source of motivation for me.

I deeply appreciate Emma O'Connor's contribution as co-author of Chapter 24: Body Image, Healthy at Any Weight and for shedding light on a valuable alternative to prioritizing a certain body image as the epitome of beauty. Emma, thank you for your contributions as a nutrition graduate student intern from North Carolina Central University.

A special thanks to the Get Published Now team. Your guidance and expertise have been invaluable throughout this process. Your support has been key in bringing this book to life and ensuring it reaches those who need it most.

Finally, I would like to give a special nod to my late husband, Jacob Opper. Jake, you always reminded me of the value this work brings into the world when you said, "You are saving lives." Your belief in me and continued support has been a guiding light, and your spirit continues to inspire me every day.

With heartfelt gratitude,

Kay

Endnotes

1: Hall, Kevin D, Kahan, Scott. Maintenance of Lost Weight and Long-Term Management of Obesity. Medical Clinics of North America. 2018 Jan;102(1):183-197. doi: 10.1016/j.mcna.2017.08.012. PMID: 29156185; PMCID: PMC5764193.

2: Van Der Kolk, Bessel. *The Body Keeps the Score: Brain, Mind, and Boy in the Healing of Trauma.* Penguin Books. 2015. p. 57.

3: See Hall and Kahan.

4: Khubchandani J, Price JH, Sharma S, Wiblishauser MJ, Webb FJ. COVID-19 pandemic and weight gain in American adults: A nationwide population-based study. Diabetes Metab Syndr. 2022 Jan;16(1):102392. doi: 10.1016/j.dsx.2022.102392. Epub 2022 Jan 10. PMID: 35030452; PMCID: PMC8743853.

5: Juul F, Parekh N, Martinez-Steele E, Monteiro CA, Chang VW. Ultra-processed food consumption among US adults from 2001 to 2018. Am J Clin Nutr. 2022 Jan 11;115(1):211-221. doi: 10.1093/ajcn/nqab305. PMID: 34647997.

6: Centers for Disease Control. "Adult Obesity Facts." May 17, 2022. https://www.cdc.gov/obesity/data/adult.html.

7: Centers for Disease Control. "Long-term Trends in Diabetes." April 2017. https://www.cdc.gov/diabetes/data/.

8: Later editions of Habits Not Diets: The Secret to Lifetime Weight Control by James M. Ferguson and Cassandra Ferguson can be found, published by Bull Publishing Company.

9: Hardy, Darren. *The Compound Effect: Jumpstart Your Income, Your Life, Your Success.* Hachette Go. 2020.

10: Clear, James. *Atomic Habits: An Easy and Proven Way to Build Good Habits and Break Bad Ones.* Random House Business Books. 2015. p. 27.

11: Thich Nhat Han. *How to Love.* Parallax Press. 2014.

12: You can find a full list of client stories for you to reference at the end of this book.

13: Brewer JA, Davis JH, Goldstein J. Why is it so hard to pay attention, or is it? Mindfulness, the factors of awakening and reward-based learning. Mindfulness (N Y). 2013 Mar 1;4(1):10.1007/s12671-012-0164-8. doi: 10.1007/s12671-012-0164-8. PMID: 24244224; PMCID: PMC3827730.

14: Dweck, Carol. *Mindset: The New Psychology of Success*. Ballantine Books. 2007.

15: Hendricks, Gay. *The Joy of Genius: The Next Step Beyond the Big Leap—a New Way to End Negative Thinking and Liberate Your True Creativity*. Waterside Productions. 2018.

16: Kushner, Robert and Nancy Kushner. *Dr. Kushner's Personality Type Diet*. St. Martin's Griffin. 2004.

17: Seligman, Martin. *Flourish: A Visionary New Understanding of Happiness and Well-being*. Atria Books. 2012.

18: Pink, Daniel. *Drive: The Surprising Truth About What Motivates Us*. Riverhead Books. 2011.

19: *Atomic Habits*, p. 65.

20: *Atomic Habits*, p. 198.

21: Kagan, Robert and Lisa Laskow Lahey. *Immunity to Change, How to Overcome it and Unlock the Potential in Yourself and Your Organization*. Harvard Business Review Press. 2009.

22: *Immunity to Change*, p. 50.

23: Lucas, Meghan. *Dear Strong Woman, You Make the Rules: How to Rewrite the Rules You Live By, So You can Live Life on Your Terms*. 2022.

24: Dalai Lama, Desmond Tutu, and Douglas Abrams. *The Book of Joy: Lasting Happiness in a Changing World*. Avery. 2016.

25: American Psychological Association. "Stress in America 2022: Concerned for the future, beset by inflation." October 2022. https://www.apa.org/news/press/releases/stress/2022/concerned-future-inflation.

26: Cross, Rob and Karen Dillon. "The Hidden Toll of Microstress." *Harvard Business Review*. February 7, 2023. https://hbr.org/2023/02/the-hidden-toll-of-microstress.

27: American Academy of Sleep Medicine. "Seven or more hours of sleep per night: A health necessity for adults." June 1, 2015. https://aasm.org/seven-or-more-hours-of-sleep-per-night-a-health-necessity-for-adults/.

28: Papatriantafyllou, E, Efthymiou, D, Zoumbaneas, E, Popescu, CA. Sleep Deprivation: Effects on Weight Loss and Weight Loss Maintenance. Nutrients. 2022, 14, 1549. https://doi.org/10.3390/nu14081549.

29: Marina Khidekel. *Your Time to Thrive, End Burnout, increase well-being and unlock your Full Potential with the New Science of Microsteps*. Hachette Go. 2021.

30: Adams, Marilee. *Change Your Questions, Change Your Life, 10 Powerful Tools for Life and Work.* Berrett-Koehler Publishers. 2009.

31: Dominick, Heather. Different. 2024. Learn more at differentthebook.com.

32: Hamilton, Diane. *Cracking the Curiosity Code: The Key to Unlocking Human Potential.* 2019.

33: Skinner, BF. *Walden Two.* Hackett Publishing Company, Inc. 2005.

34: Sun Y, Rong S, Liu B, Du Y, Wu Y, Chen L, Xiao Q, Snetselaar L, Wallace R, Bao W. Meal Skipping and Shorter Meal Intervals Are Associated with Increased Risk of All-Cause and Cardiovascular Disease Mortality among US Adults. J Acad Nutr Diet. 2023 Mar;123(3):417-426.e3. doi: 10.1016/j.jand.2022.08.119. Epub 2022 Aug 11. PMID: 35964910.

35: This segment from *The Today Show* aired on August 15, 2023. At the time of publishing, you can view it at https://www.today.com/video/sheryl-lee-ralph-shares-life-advice-surprises-deserving-teacher-190857797649.

36: Canfield, Jack. *The Success Principles: How to Get from Where You Are to Where You Want to Be.* Mariner Books. 2015.

37: Transcript of author's interview with Jack Canfield. April 6, 2022.

38: Murthy, Vivek. Posted on his facebook page on April 21, 2017. https://www.facebook.com/DrVivekMurthy/posts/251023231970308.

39: Kay, Katty and Claire Shipman. *The Confidence Code: The Science and Art of Self Assurance, What Every Woman Should Know.* Harper Business. 2018.

40: Murakami, Haruki. *What I Talk About When I Talk About Running.* Knopf Doubleday Publishing Group. 2009.

41: Chodron, Pema. *Start Where You Are: A Guide to Compassionate Living.* Shambhala. 2018.

42: Brach, Tara. *Radical Compassion, Learning to Love Yourself and Your World with the Practice of RAIN.* Penguin Life. 2020.

43: Salzberg, Sharon. "The Myth of Multitasking" in *Real Happiness at Work: Meditations for Accomplishment, Achievement, and Peace.* Workman Publishing Company. 2013.

44: For more information about research about the health effects of the Mediterranean Diet visit https://www.nhlbi.nih.gov/news/2020/researchers-explore-link-between-mediterranean-diet-and-health.

45: For more information about the DASH eating plan visit https://www.nhlbi.nih.gov/education/dash/following-dash

46: To learn more about making better dietary choices, go to the Dietary Guidelines for Americans, 2020-2025 Report at https://www.dietaryguidelines.gov/. For other eating tips, visit https://www.myplate.gov/.

47: Learn more at https://health.gov/our-work/nutrition-physical-activity/phys-ical-activity-guidelines/current-guidelines/top-10-things-know. Visit https://health.gov/our-work/nutrition-physical-activity/move-your-way-communi-ty-resources/campaign-materials/materials-adults#videos for fact sheets, posters and videos for more ideas about how to fit more physical activity into your life. See also: https://health.gov/moveyourway.

48: Learn more at https://www.nhlbi.nih.gov/health/educational/lose_wt/recom-men.htm#:~:text=Weight%20loss%20should%20be%20about,practical%20way%20to%20reduce%20calories.

49: Wansink, Brian. *Mindless Eating: Why We Eat More Than We Think.* Bantam. 2007.

50: The Food Industry Association. Accessed 5/14/24 at https://www.fmi.org/our-research/food-industry-facts.

51: Learn more at https://www.fda.gov/food/nutrition-facts-label/how-understand-and-use-nutrition-facts-label.

52: Mahan, L. K., & Raymond, J. L. (2017). *Krause's Food & the Nutrition Care Process* (14th ed.). Elsevier.

53: National Weight Control Registry. Downloaded 5/14/24 at http://www.nwcr.ws.

54: Intergovernmental Panel on Climate Change. *Synthesis Report of the IPCC Sixth Assessment Report (AR6) Summary for Policymakers.* Intergovernmental Panel on Climate Change; 2023. https://www.ipcc.ch/report/ar6/syr/downloads/report/IPCC_AR6_SYR_SPM.pdf

55: Crippa M, Solazzo E, Guizzardi D, Monforti-Ferrario F, Tubiello FN, Leip A. Food Systems Are Responsible for a Third of Global Anthropogenic GHG Emissions. *Nature Food.* 2021

56: P. Edwards and I Roberts. 2009. Population adiposity and climate change. International Journal of Epidemiology published online by Oxford University Press, doi:10.1093/ije/dyp172 and downloaded on April 25, 2014 at http://ije.oxfordjournals.org/content/38/4/1137.abstract?sid=5a811782-7bd7-4275-a2d3-4fd8c2fdbbff.

57: For more, see United Nations," Food and Climate Change: Healthy diets for a healthier planet," at: https://www.un.org/en/climatechange/science/climate-issues/food.

58: G. Eshel and P. A. Martin. 2006. "Diet, energy, and global warming." *Earth Interactions* 10(9): 1-17.

59: *Mindless Eating.*

60: USDA, Economic Research Service. Food Consumption Up 16 Percent Since 1970. November 1, 2005. The ERS food consumption (per capita) data series, one of the few series tracking long-term consumption. Downloaded on 1/27/24 at https://www.ers.usda.gov/data-products/food-availability-per-capita-data-system/.

61: UN News Ref: Once Again U.S. and Europe Way Ahead on Daily Caloric Intake, Dec. 12, 2022. Downloaded 1/26/24 at: https://news.un.org/en/story/2022/12/1131637.

62: National Library of Medicine, National Institutes of Health. Restaurant Food Consumption by US Adults. FSRG Dietary Data Brief No. 48. Downloaded on 1/27/24 at: https://www.ncbi.nlm.nih.gov/books/NBK588579/?report=printable

63: David Kessler, *The End of Overeating: Taking Control of the Insatiable American Appetite*, Rodale, 2009.

64: NIH, NIDDK, Overweight & Obesity Statistics. Downloaded on Jan. 27, 2024 https://www.niddk.nih.gov/health-information/health-statistics/overweight-obesity#prevalence.

65: C B, Martin, et al. CDC, National Center for Health Statistics. Attempts to Lose Weight Among Adults in the United States, 2013-2016. NCHS Data Brief No. 313, July 2018. Downloaded on 1/27/24 https://www.cdc.gov/nchs/products/databriefs/db313.htm#:~:text=Nearly%20one%2Dhalf%20(49.1%25),40%E2%80%9359%20(52.4%25).

66: Ward, Z, Bleich S., Long M, et al. Association of body mass index with health care expenditures in the United States by age and ses. Plos One. 2021. Downloaded on 1/27/24 at: https://journals.plos.org/plosone/article?id=10.1371/journal.pone.0247307

67: OECD. *Policy Insights.*; 2017. https://www.oecd.org/els/health-systems/Obesity-Update-2017.pdf.

About the Author

KAY LOUGHREY, nutrition expert, weight loss coach, and speaker, has helped herself and hundreds of adults lose weight and maintain the weight loss. She began her nutrition and weight loss company in 2012 after a 27-year career in public health where she helped Americans adopt healthier lifestyle choices. Kay is a nutritionist and dietitian with a Master of Public Health degree in nutrition who offers adults real solutions to weight loss struggles. Kay who lives in the Maryland suburbs of Washington, DC, loves good food and travel and has taken more than 20 trips to favorite destinations in Europe (France, Italy, Switzerland, Austria, Croatia, Poland, and the Czech Republic) and the Caribbean.

To receive access to your Companion Guidebook visit: visit https://www.sweetlifewellness.com/guidebook/

www.ingramcontent.com/pod-product-compliance
Lightning Source LLC
Chambersburg PA
CBHW070103030426
42335CB00016B/1989